NURSING ROLES

SERIES ON NURSING ADMINISTRATION

EDITORS

SONA

SERIES ON NURSING ADMINISTRATION

An annual publication planned and administered by the University of Iowa, SONA addresses current and emerging issues in nursing administration. In each volume, distinguished nurse administrators and educators address the state of knowledge, future directions, and controversial questions on aspects of a particular issue and propose options for resolution. The series provides a quality resource for practicing administrators, faculty teaching nursing administration, and students in administration programs.

NURSING ROLES
Evolving or Recycled?

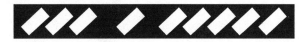

Sue Moorhead
Editor

Diane Gardner Huber
Chair of the Board

SONA 9

Series on Nursing Administration

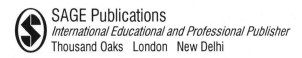

SAGE Publications
International Educational and Professional Publisher
Thousand Oaks   London   New Delhi

For information address:

SAGE Publications, Inc.
2455 Teller Road
Thousand Oaks, California 91320
E-mail: order@sagepub.com

SAGE Publications Ltd.
6 Bonhill Street
London EC2A 4PU
United Kingdom

SAGE Publications India Pvt. Ltd.
M-32 Market
Greater Kailash I
New Delhi 110 048 India

Printed in the United States of America

Library of Congress Cataloging-in-Publication Data

Main entry under title:

Nursing roles: evolving or recycled? / editor, Sue Moorhead.
    p. cm. — (Series on nursing administration; v. 9)
    Includes bibliographical references and index.
    ISBN 0-7619-0149-3
    1. Nursing specialties. 2. Nurse practitioners. 3. Nursing—
Vocational guidance. I. Moorhead, Sue. II. Series.
RT86.7.N94 1997
610.73′069—dc20   96-35619

97 98 99 00 01 02 03 10 9 8 7 6 5 4 3 2 1

Acquiring Editor:	Daniel Ruth
Editorial Assistant:	Jessica Crawford
Production Editor:	Michele Lingre
Production Assistant:	Sherrise Purdum
Typesetter/Designer:	Janelle LeMaster
Indexer:	Cristina Haley
Cover Designer:	Lesa Valdez

As the final steps in the publication of this 9th volume of SONA
were underway, news of Kathy Kelly's sudden death shocked
those of us intimately involved in the publication of this series.
Kathy Kelly served as the editor of Volumes 5 through 8 of SONA
and received the AJN Book of the Year Award for Volume 6 titled,
Health Care Rationing: Dilemma and Paradox. She was a member
of the Editorial Board since its inception. Her patience, support,
enthusiasm, and dedication to high standards for this publication
were unending. It is appropriate that this volume focusing on
the changing roles for nursing be dedicated in her memory.

She is greatly missed by her colleagues and students.

❖ ❖ ❖

Contents

Series Preface

Today's nurse executive needs to stay current in many rapidly changing areas of health care. To meet this demand, the **Series on Nursing Administration** is designed to give nursing administrators new information on current and emerging issues. Developed and managed at the University of Iowa College of Nursing and published by Sage Publications, Inc., it is a quality resource for nurse executives, faculty who teach nursing administration, and students in nursing administration programs. Each year a new volume addresses the most recent issues in this discipline. Thus, a subscription to the series will keep readers on the forefront of knowledge and practice.

Every nurse executive interacts with corporate management; colleagues in other settings, professional groups, the community, and clients; and with nurse colleagues, members of other disciplines, and ancillary personnel. To stay current with developments in each of these areas, the nurse executive reads journals and newsletters, attends continuing education programs, and participates in short-term executive management courses. The most effective method, however, is sharing concerns, experiences, and insights with peers. The Sage **Series on Nursing Administration** formalizes the process of sharing among experts with similar concerns. In every chapter of each volume of the series, expert authors share their experiences and ideas on particular emerging issues. Busy nurse executives can conveniently and cost-effectively keep their knowledge current on a variety of topics by reading this series.

Nursing administration faculty can use the series to keep their teaching and practice alive, current, and timely. Most nursing administration programs have one or more courses that address issues in nursing management. Because these issues undergo rapid change, faculty need a flexible approach to teaching this content. This series offers the instructor maximum flexibility in selecting issues for discussion to fit the needs of a particular class. An instructor teaching a nursing management issues course can use the series as a course text. Students introduced to this series will find it a resource with ongoing value. Faculty teaching undergraduate level administration courses also can use the series to supplement an introductory text on management and leadership.

This series is unique in that it is the first annual series devoted to issues in nursing administration. To ensure that it covers current issues and provides up-to-date information, the series employs a unique publication process involving four groups: a series editor, an editorial board, the authors, and the publisher.

The editor of Volumes 1 to 4 of the series is Marion Johnson, RN, PhD, an associate professor at the University of Iowa. She has a rich practice base in nursing administration and currently teaches nursing administration at the master's level. Her background, interests, and writing skills made her eminently qualified for the job of series editor.

Kathleen Kelly, PhD, RN, was editor for Volumes 5 to 8 of the series. Kathleen had years of experience as a community health nursing administrator and taught nursing administration at the master's level. She also administers the Continuing Education Program at the College of Nursing. Her work pro- vides a broad perspective on issues that are of critical importance to nurse executives and managers.

Sue Moorhead, PhD, RN, is editor starting with Volume 9. Sue has years of experience in administration as a U.S. Army nurse and currently is an assistant professor at the University of Iowa. The military provided her with a diverse clinical background and a broad perspective of administrative issues in nursing. She currently teaches undergraduate students at the College of Nursing.

The editorial board consists of faculty teaching in the nursing administration program at Iowa and selected nurse administrators associated with the program. The board meets three to four times a year with the series editor, helps identify the emerging issues and prospective authors, and assists the editor with manuscript review. Iowa's growing program in nursing administration, including study at the doctoral level, makes this an ideal setting to support this publication. A National Advisory Board consisting of nursing administrators, both academic and practicing, advises the editorial board on pertinent topics and authors where needed.

The authors are distinguished nurse administrators, educators, and researchers chosen for their expertise in particular areas. Although authors have the freedom to pursue an issue as they choose, each is encouraged to address the state of knowledge, future directions, and the controversial questions surrounding the issue, and to propose one or more options for resolution. Beginning with Volume 7, authors were chosen by a review process following a Call for Abstracts. The Call for Abstracts is mailed and advertised in various journals and newsletters during the months of February through September each year.

The publisher of the series, beginning with volume VII, is Sage Publications, Inc. Mosby-Year Book, Inc. published Volumes III to VI, and Volumes I and II were published by Addison-Wesley.

All of us involved in this series believe that it will benefit not only those who teach and practice nursing administration but the entire nursing profession, and most important, the patients we serve. We welcome your comments and suggestions.

—Diane Gardner Huber, PhD, RN
Chairperson, Editorial Board, Volumes 9–11

—Meridean Maas, PhD, RN, FAAN
Chairperson, Editorial Board, Volumes 5–8

—Joanne Comi McCloskey, PhD, RN, FAAN
Chairperson, Editorial Board, Volumes 1–4

Introduction

The ninth volume of the **Series on Nursing Administration** (SONA) explores the changing roles of nurses in today's rapidly fluctuating health care environment. This volume offers the reader a wide range of potential roles for nurses and captures the complexity and diversity of nursing in the present health care arena. Some roles discussed in this volume are new and are evolving from the issues and challenges in the health care delivery system. Other chapters present roles that, for those of us who have been nurses for a while, seem familiar and yet changed since our first encounter. This volume of SONA captures the variety of roles nurses perform today. The ability of nurses to redefine and change their professional roles during times of health care reform is perhaps nursing's greatest asset and the key to survival as a profession.

In the first chapter of this volume, Koerner and Burgess challenge nurses to abandon old mindsets about practice that are no longer useful and to develop professional values and beliefs about the delivery and outcomes of health care that will provide the process and structure needed for the present chaotic health care system. They argue that the future requires nurses to focus on care coordination, client education, and an approach to quality outcomes that uses teams of health care providers in an interdependent effort across the continuum of care. This chapter provides a thought-provoking overview of the roles for nurses today and in the future.

In Chapter 2, Erlen discusses the ethical issues nurse administrators face as they attempt to reconcile the competing goals of quality patient care with the fiscal management of the organization in a managed care environment. Ethical issues such as privacy of the patient, advocating quality care, acting in a just manner, challenging institutional policies and practices, and fostering organizational integrity are included. Erlen advocates that nurse administrators need to examine both new and reframed ethical questions to balance the goals of quality patient care with those of the organization. The discussion of possible ways to deal with these issues provides insight to nurse administrators dealing with the managed care environment in health care.

The rapid changes in the health care arena have created new opportunities for nurses as entrepreneurs who deliver new services and products. In Chapter 3, Redman examines entrepreneurship, its implications for nursing, and the opportunities, risks, and challenges it offers for nurses. This role for nurses provides autonomy and flexibility in ways that have not existed in health care organizations in the past. This discussion of entrepreneurship is helpful for nurses considering a business venture as a new career option.

In Chapter 4, Helms and Anderson provide an overview of the five-step policy process of agenda setting, analysis, decision making, implementation, and evaluation. Understanding policy allows nurses to consider the multiple factors that affect the policy process, such as timing, resources, social and organizational interaction, preferences, culture, and luck. The authors discuss the tendency for policy to have long periods of stability and incremental policy making, then occasional rapid and radical shifts in policy approaches. The application of the policy process to the emerging health care system provides insight and a useful approach for nurses.

An evolving role that has developed rapidly as a response to technology in health care is the informatics nurse. In Chapter 5, Delaney, Mehmert, and Johnson discuss the historical development of this role, the characteristics and competencies of informatics nurses, and the role of this specialty in changing health care. The authors provide useful information for nurse administrators regarding the effective management of the evolving role of the informatics nurse.

Two chapters in this volume focus on the use of unlicensed assistive personnel as a solution to some of the problems faced in a cost-conscious health care environment. In Chapter 6, Deckert, Friend, and MacDonald describe one hospital's efforts to redesign the work of nurses. This redesign effort created the need for assistance by unlicensed assistive personnel. The authors relate their experiences with this planned change in their organization.

Afifi describes another strategy for using unlicensed personnel in health care delivery. Today, nurses are faced with many problems related to access to care for specific cultural groups and the need to deliver culturally relevant care. One strategy, the use of an indigenous health worker, is described in Chapter 7. The strategy uses unlicensed personnel as either employees or volunteers and depends on a team approach in which the nurse is assisted by an indigenous health worker to enhance care. This approach results in increased access to services, increased compliance to prescribed treatments, and improved outcomes of care using cultural beliefs, language, and appropriate methods for the group. The predictions for a more culturally diverse population in the United States over the next half century will require nurse administrators to deal with issues related to providing culturally sensitive health care as a component of quality care.

In this volume, two chapters address models of nursing practice. In Chapter 8, Daly describes the Life Care Nursing Model used to provide care to older adults living in both independent living apartments or within the care facility of a midwestern retirement residence. Outcomes for the nursing staff and residents are evaluated based on care provided with this model. In Chapter 9, Tappan and colleagues also describe a project designed to test an innovative model of nursing practice. The chapter critically analyzes the issues and strategies that were encountered with nurses making the transition from inpatient care to community-based care. The insights from using these models will be helpful to nurse administrators contemplating similar nursing role changes in their organization.

The final four chapters in this volume are devoted to advanced practice roles. It is clear that advanced practice is an area that is expanding and evolving at a rapid pace in nursing. In Chapter 10, Harrison discusses the role of advanced practice nurses as hospitals transition into a managed-care environment. Key contributions provided by nurses in advanced practice are decreased acute-care use rates, shortened length of hospital stays, and improved patient outcomes. In Chapter 11, Haddock describes the third generation clinical nurse specialist and advocates for nurse administrators to support these nurses as they transition into either nurse practitioner or case manager roles to meet the need of patients in the present health care environment. In Chapter 12, Norsen and colleagues describe the acute care nurse practitioner role as important for the future because it addresses the complex needs of patients. The authors elaborate on this role using the Strong Model of Advanced Practice. The final chapter of Volume 9 by Walker and Sebastian focuses on the acute care nurse practitioner and nurse care manager roles for improving the care of patients with chronic illness. The authors describe how these two advanced practice roles complement each other to address the care of patients requiring frequent use of health care services.

Each chapter of this volume describes an important role of nurses in today's health care arena. The authors describe the development, characteristics or the role, and its relevance to nursing's future. Health care providers, managers and administrators, educators, and researchers will benefit from examining current roles in nursing and the experiences of other nurses in this era of rapid change in health care.

Sue Moorhead, PhD, RN

CHAPTER 1

Nursing's Role and Functions in a Seamless Continuum of Care

JoEllen Koerner
Constance S. Burgess

In this chaotic era of health care restructuring, all organizations and health professions, including nursing, are called to reexamine their strategy, structure, and function activities as professional roles are changing and evolving. We must move beyond well-defined organizational boundaries and autonomous professional roles to a more inclusive focus on process, purpose, and people working together in an interdisciplinary fashion with the patient central to the work. As we redesign geographical, functional, and relational boundaries and processes, nursing will facilitate individuals, groups, and society in moving toward a new reality of health.

The new health care paradigm hears and heeds messages given by professionals who speak in a clear and active voice. If we as nurses are to be credible participants in shaping the future of health care and our own destiny, clarity in our communications to one another and to others is imperative. The customary convention for professional publications is for authors to remain in the passive third person and heavily reference existing literature. Because this chapter reflects the authors' shared opinions that have risen out of a collection of national experiences, exposures, and conversations, we have chosen to speak in the active first person to our colleagues in the field.

1

Health care is spinning in a chaotic frenzy as old structures and forms are falling apart. In this time of new economic imperatives, health care professionals have been called upon to reexamine their practices, professional values, and beliefs about the delivery and outcomes of health care in general, while enlarging their focus on wellness and rehabilitation services. The new health care paradigm demands extraordinary expertise, phenomenal creativity, a command of finance and information systems, mastery of managed care principles, and a great sense of humor.

Leland Kaiser observed that the only security you have in a time of chaos is yourself... the essence of who you are and what you can bring to any situation (1995). This is also true of nursing, a profession as old as humankind. The current debate about what is and is not nursing is timely and essential as the profession crafts its place in the emerging new order. If nurses are to be viable and powerful players in the health care field, what will ensure their space is being *relevant* to the needs of society—continuing to have something essential to contribute in life-giving ways. This calls the discipline members to reconsider the assumptions and beliefs held dear about who they are and what their role offers. Nurses must reframe their roles and their work to fit the emerging new reality.

This chapter explores the philosophical parameters affecting nursing roles in times of change and redesign. Nurses' roles must be adapted to a changing society that is increasingly becoming more diverse and chronically ill. Further, the isolated institution model is giving way to an integrated continuum, and nurses' work space is expanding; wherever there are people, there is a place for nursing in preventative, primary, or supportive roles. The prevailing autonomous view in all professions must give way to an interdependent one that demands a high degree of collaboration and cooperation. Finally, the notion of client as passive recipient of care from an expert professional fades when we view individuals as experts in their own health and the health care system as a vehicle to support them in their efforts to maximize their life journey in the health experience.

REFRAMING OUR BELIEFS

Assumptions are simply beliefs that frame our reality. Individuals make assumptions because they create the reality one claims. Realities are not right or wrong ... they simply *are*. It is our reality frame that maintains security because it gives definition to phenomenon and provides guidance for decisions to be made. A changing reality evokes fear and resistance because it requires new ways of thinking and being in the world. Once we experience something new, we cannot return to the old way. Our circle of reality has enlarged . . . and so has our responsibility.

Held assumptions can be discerned by listening to what people say. The way one uses words reflects the way one thinks, and thinking reflects assumptions. If we listen closely to the nursing dialogue, there is reason for concern. Closer examination of current nursing literature reflects:

1. Patients come to the hospital to receive nursing care
2. Nurses alone can do many of the technical tasks required in hospital and home settings . . . it is the foundational work of nursing
3. Strategies to reduce costs and increase productivity disregard quality for the patient
4. By reducing the number of services provided to patients, the care is marginalized
5. Autonomy in nursing practice is a primary value for the discipline
6. Nursing must maintain its place at "the table"
7. Nursing is at risk because of outside forces

This list is offset by a growing theme in the literature demonstrating exciting programs and practices that are moving forward in concert with the challenges found in the field. Unfortunately, however, the stated list reflects many concerns about nursing that are all too frequently brought to redesign tables set by decision makers focusing more broadly on the client, payor, the aggregate of providers—nurse, physician, therapists, social workers—and an empowered consumer. Unless collective nursing broadens its view of the emerging reality and reframes the profession's essential core essence in new and relevant roles and processes, it will be left behind. We believe more appropriate and pertinent assumptions might be

1. Clients come to a hospital and other service settings to receive comprehensive care based on their presenting needs
2. The art and science of nursing practice is a process that facilitates individual choices and activities that increase the value and quality of people's lives
3. The driving force for change in health care is managed care with a focus on reimbursement management because of decreasing resources coupled with increasing demand for services
4. There must be a connection between professional ideology and real world practice
5. The risks to nurses are equal to those of every other discipline, no more and no less; therefore, the opportunities are also equal
6. The real enemy to nursing lies within the discipline because of outdated assumptions coupled with this attitude: We "eat our young" and "shoot our old" (wisdom keepers and leaders)

A key redesign principle states that excellence eliminates competition. If you are practicing the state of the art, no one can replace you. Nursing—*and all disciplines*—have been given a "wake-up" call. Each discipline is called to reframe its *essential* contribution, while noting areas of shared expertise as well as gaps in service. As we redefine the important and unique contributions we hold for health and healing, we will provide a strong foundation for care in the emerging delivery pattern for a managed care environment. As we focus on the client instead of the nurse, the fears and risks to the discipline will be minimized because our contribution will be essential to high-quality, low-cost care. We can then sit at the multiple tables set for reform debate and present our contribution while partnering in new ways with others in the industry.

REALIGNING OUR FOCUS

In every moment lies all potential possibility. The reality we experience is the one we create by the things we focus on. The health care world—in *all* professional disciplines—comprises reformers and transformers. Reformers, who try to control the process of change, hold themselves away from the emerging reality, judging it from the outside. They offer criticism and take the role of victim based on outmoded models of understanding. Reformers memorize and adhere to other people's thoughts and fears, believing that if they (nurses) cooperate with the changes, they will be overrun by powerful "others." They can see all the difficulties, challenges, and potential losses a change of such magnitude would take. Reformers want things in their image, they cannot understand intellectually the evolutionary opportunity that lies in a transformative moment; this must come from within rather than from outside (Small, 1992).

Transformers, on the other hand, come to a new way of thinking. They focus on conditions of health rather than symptoms of disease. Process, pattern, vision, paradox, and flow replace the outworn emphasis on specific events, outward form, and manipulation of parts. Holistic healing, intuition, warmth, love, and collaboration replace diagnostics, labeling, testing, prescribing, and controlling. These practitioners (nurses) carry a consciousness that gently, confidently invites others to break out of old stereotypes and risk becoming themselves. The essence of all people, provider and client alike, is toward creation, expansion, inclusiveness, and spontaneity. Care delivery models and practices that are built on these principles will bring society closer to experiencing the qualities of being human and whole.

Nursing's essential charge to assist others toward health and wholeness or experience a good death emanates from our history. This has been done in an environment that held moderate complexity and diversity, moving at a gentle and predictable pace. As we move into the end of an era, all major institutions and ideologies woefully lack structures and processes to adequately address the multifaceted and rapidly changing needs of society. By moving and focusing only on things that served us well in the past, we quickly sound and act in antiquated ways as we address the much broader needs of multiple constituencies in the health care arena.

Although some nurse leaders are crafting new models for patient care delivery, many nursing executives focus on saving traditional hospital-based nursing because they cannot see the bigger picture. Nursing practice in these settings translates into a continued energizing and highlighting of the technical side of nursing, whereas the more complex professional processes of the discipline flounder, or continue unnoticed and unclaimed. Focusing on nursing as an autonomous profession rather than as an essential player in an interdependent team misses the richness of relationship with our health care colleagues. Further, and more dangerously, it negates the integrative and coordinative role that institutional nursing—the 24-hour presence at the bedside—provides for the entire health care team. This integrative focus beyond institutional borders can and must be addressed by nursing case management models for the complex chronicity that now resides in the community. When nursing leaders create a "report card" for nursing that holds nurses—in isolation—accountable for things they do with or on behalf of an entire care team, nursing has been placed in an unfeasible situation.

Advanced practice nurses caught in the traditional mindset continue to say, "I am the Clinical Nurse Specialist or Nurse Practitioner, this is what I do," whereas the health care payor is asking "What is it that we and the client need and who is best to meet that need?" Reformers continue to speak of who and what they are, never seeing that essentially those things may—or may not—meet the pressing needs of the person or the organization. Transformers with the capacity for astute listening and reflective practice skills ask the more appropriate question, "Given this situation, what is essential, what part of it can I provide uniquely and what part requires the services of a comprehensive team?" This practitioner then draws together appropriate players and services so they can create a comprehensive plan that addresses the care needs of the specific client, based on what the client deems as essential for her or her own well-being.

Staff nurses also can be caught in a focus that is too small. These nurses will cling tenaciously to the tasks they have done for years. Their focus on skill acquisition around equipment and protocol management is an outgrowth of the technological era that swept our nation in the 1960s and 1970s as a result of the U.S. space program. Institutions across America established intensive care units and multiple services based on the most advanced equipment and supplies available in the world. Nursing, in its honorable tradition, quickly mastered the use and application of these devices on behalf of client care. Although this is still a valued part of our work, several major advances make it permissible, essential even, for professionals to delegate some of the task assignment to others. Technology now monitors and reports expert assessments that used to be done by the practitioner. Growing numbers of the well-informed public want and expect active involvement in the management of their own health. When nursing expands its focus beyond the task level, a myriad of other needs emerge because of shortened length-of-stay and chronicity among some of our client population. Delegation frees us for some of the more complex and demanding work of care coordination, client education, and facilitation of quality outcomes for a team of providers. Herein lies the new application for nursing process in the evolving health care field.

Nursing education is another arena that is challenged in this rapidly changing environment. Nursing education continues to move into the academic settings, severing formal connection to the service setting. This provided the necessary separation of education from service, and positioned nursing as an academic science-based discipline. With the increasing complexity of the health care field, several things make this model increasingly narrow. Nurse educators who had their last formal clinical experience several years ago have no current mental models that give "real-life" examples to students. These nurse educators also may not have the skills to adequately supervise students on the unit. This reality offers an opportunity for schools and service settings to partner in creation of joint-practice models that invite experienced clinicians to assume this role. Another answer might be to institute a faculty practice program, providing faculty with an active practice as well as an academic role.

Having students come into the highly acute complex medical center for most of their clinical experience exposes them to such extreme pathology that they do not experience exposure to health and chronicity in a way that gives students an experiential bank on which to make comparisons in their own practice. Moving more education into health clinics, schools, and long-term care facilities will be essential to prepare students for the emerging work environment. Finally, the new order calls for critical thinking skills and the capacity to participate in quality management teams and other groups effectively. Students must be given more opportunity for reflective rather than prescriptive thinking. Students should also become partners in designing and evaluating their unique learning experience, much as staff nurses become co-designers and managers of their unit in a shared governance model. This broader focus in the educational experience will reunite education and service in ways that are synergistic and mutually advantageous.

Nursing role redefinition must expand beyond a more comprehensive list of activities to an *enlarged focus* on public needs and nursing skill sets. In all nursing arenas, role redefinition is enhanced by a broader frame of reference that thinks in more inclusive ways. Most people are not aware that they have reality frames that are not comprehensive because it is the reality they have always known. Thus, redesign must start every conversation with the queries "Is there another way of looking at this?" "How much need is manifest here?" "Do I have all the resources essential to meet the need?" "What other resources are available?" As the focus enlarges to be more inclusive, lines that served well in the past will be redrawn . . . or removed. The larger nursing's reality becomes, the more resources the discipline will have at their disposal on behalf of quality care. The expanded vision of clinicians, academicians, and students will enlarge the value for the system and the people it serves.

REMAPPING NURSING'S CARE ENVIRONMENT

If role activity is to be congruous with societal needs, the reality of a managed care environment must be examined, noting the subtle differences between it and the traditional fee-for-service model. An increasingly diverse, well-informed public with access to increasingly sophisticated technology that is very user friendly must also be acknowledged. Finally, other nontraditional health care services with rich and varied contributions must be available for a diverse client population with differing needs displayed at various stages of their illness/wellness experience.

America launched into a socialized form of health care for citizens older than 65 with the introduction of Medicare in the 1960s. Through the years, Medicare has grown in size and scope. Long-range projections demonstrate that the aging of America will soon create a demand that cannot be sustained. Population and migration trends further enrich our society, while increasing use of health care services. As the United States becomes a more diverse and larger population living in a geographically bounded nation, issues of crime, violence, and poverty continue to rise. A radical reform in health care services is essential if we are going to maintain the health and well-being of this nation.

The face of America is multifaceted and regionally unique. Thus, health reform essentially may be a state and local phenomenon. The Canadian government has determined that it cannot create health reform globally, announcing that it must occur at the local and regional level (Kaiser, 1995). In our nation, state-generated enabling legislation that would require reform to occur at the local level is beginning to supersede any national mandate for health care reform. As nursing more closely examines the complexity of its work, this direction appears to be a prudent one.

The complexity that must be carefully addressed in role redefinition and system redesign is a major focus of administrative teams in health care systems. Murphy (1995) completed a five-year study on hospital work-redesign that encompassed 135 hospitals and more than 200,000 employees. His work demonstrated a complexity factor 2,000 times greater in health care than in any major Fortune 500 company. Further, he found that a simple takeout of 4% "across the board" increased the likelihood of negative client outcomes by 200%. He concluded with the observation that such indiscriminate redesign makes an organization as culpable for adverse client outcomes as a malpracticing physician (Murphy, 1995). Nurse executives intuitively know this and balk when they receive a decree "we must cut our costs by 15%" as a mandate versus as a target. Only when corporate goals are established based on *need*, and the entire system is examined and realigned, can these savings be realized. The challenges facing the field in reducing costs while maintaining quality so that services can be accessible and affordable to all is no easy task.

Nurse leaders provide the social conscience around political and administrative tables in redesign and health policy discussions. The career experience that brings them to the table typically includes the role of staff nurse, where they come to know the needs of the client intimately. Many are then promoted to the position of unit director, where they learn to coordinate the needs of clients with resources provided by physicians and allied health providers within the strategic plan of the organization, standards of various professional groups and performance evaluation criteria of accrediting agencies. As they emerge into corporate or political "leader space," they come to the table with an insider's perspective and a sense of clinical process that is essential to the broad discussions surrounding health care reform and redesign.

Nursing speaks frequently about "the table." We must be placed at the corporate table, while establishing other tables that invite broad participation in decision making around strategic planning, policy, restructuring, managed care contracting, product line development, and creation of alternative delivery systems, to name a few. We do not need permission to do so. Rather, we must use the power and leverage of our positions to facilitate dialogue among the many care providers around these important issues that create the foundation for quality and cost-effective care delivery.

For nurse leaders to grow into major organizational leadership roles they must understand managed care *intimately*. It is not enough to simply comprehend costs, capitation, and so on. We must also understand incentives, strategies, long-term goals of all stakeholders; payors, employers, and providers. As we come to know and appreciate the multiple facets, motives, values, and incentives of all the stakeholders, we can provide leadership to meet those goals. Then and only then will we contribute to and potentially lead major organizational change toward building alternative delivery sites, designing systems for continuity through the continuum.

Simultaneously, the Nurse Executive must be able to articulate to the Chief Executive Officer and Executive Management Team the added value of nursing to the business. It is not sufficient to state that the organization is what it is because of excellent nursing care. We must be able to translate our services into financial outcomes, coupled with stories that illustrate the unique contribution nurses have made in their roles of facilitation and integration. Are nurses seen and experienced as strategic thinkers, planners, and marketers for the organization? Do nurses integrate their own unique fund of knowledge with the broad picture by providing information that can elevate the organization's problem-solving and planning to a higher level of quality and efficiency? Staff can only develop this level of professional and business acumen when the Nurse Executive acquires, analyzes, and communicates corporate information and strategy to the staff. Further, staff nurses need education and experiential opportunities to develop related information management skills. Their activity must be supported by integrating their work into systems designed to facilitate and capture their contribution.

REDEFINING OUR WORK AND OUR RELATIONSHIPS

Nursing's response to health care reform must be first and foremost local, based on the unique needs of the environment. Patterns and strategies are emerging nationally, but they must be adapted locally to serve the particular needs of the local market. Variables to be assessed in the process of redesign include size of community and community needs; number of employers composing their workforce, allied health services available, staff mix and human resources available, physician profile, managed care penetration, types of payment currently in place, and incentives being offered. Payor mix must be considered, identifying which are revenue producing (fee-for-service, percent discount per diem) and which are expense (case-rate, diagnosis-related groups [DRGs], capitated). They must also consider that if an organization moves too quickly, it can cut the revenue stream too soon.

These are elements nurse leaders must critically analyze as they create a strategy and timely implementation plan. Noted psychologist Emil Erikson made an observation on his 89th birthday. He added a ninth stage to his previous eight stages of development—the stage of wisdom. He observed that there have been great individuals comparable with Lincoln, Ghandi, and Eleanor Roosevelt in the past. But what made these individuals truly giants in their eras was timing. The needs of society and the ideology of these persons came into perfect alignment in such a way that they were drawn to those positions almost in spite of themselves. Erikson admonished that timing is the most critical element of wisdom that one can possess. If we are pushing too hard, or feel the hard edge of resistance too deeply, it means that people are not ready. We must simply generate ideas and the essentials needed to actualize them, recognizing the moment that they are needed. These carefully thought out and developed strategies can then be presented as an answer to an issue you know intimately—and the new way is born (Melville, 1992).

A guiding principle that *the end lies in the beginning* is foundational to good planning (Burgess, 1995). Thus, the vision created and outcomes established dictate the process undertaken. Kaiser (1995) asserted that the name of the game is a designer community, nation, and globe. Through cooperation and sharing of resources at all levels of the universe, we find abundance that is not evident in a competitive win-lose environment. We must be inclusive at the design table or the model is destined to failure. As the plan evolves from various discussion tables, players in the new arena must be supported through education and pilot projects that allow experimentation with delivery process, documentation forms, and decision-making models that are more inclusive.

Those who are powering through the American health care industry with "hostile takeover" strategies will ultimately lose the game. Those who operate from a "client-driven" agenda will adapt, flex, and provide necessary expertise to meet the needs of the client, the practitioners, and the organization. The notion that the client belongs to the nurse is an old one suggesting territorial, possessive posturing. Collective nursing must stop protecting nursing for the sake of nursing and start investing in, and being accountable to, the whole industry, primarily the client. Nursing's uniqueness will be preserved because of competence, knowledge, and skills, not because we deserve it, we powered our way there, or we are unique. Every discipline is unique to or for something. We are moving from the era of autonomy to an era of interdependence, where the collective IQ of various minds far exceeds that of any single individual. This calls for greater maturity and capacity of individual practitioners. It is this individual mental shift, not the specific role of RN, MD, and so on, that will determine which professionals will continue with careers and which will ultimately be left behind.

CARE CONTINUUM AS A PROCESS

Multidisciplinary groups are increasingly dealing with the continuum of care concept. Is it a grouping of providers in various setting throughout a geographic region that all clients move across in a prescribed fashion? Or is it a process that is created for each client based on that client's unique and pressing needs? The first is navigated through predetermined maps and protocols, the second is fueled and driven by a "salient factors" approach.

A salient factor (Burgess, 1995) is defined simply as a key issue, something striking, or something that stands out. Used in the context of client care planning, it identifies the key issues in the client's life that must be addressed before the client can return home or move to the next level of care. Salient factors look beyond the physical impairment issues and account for all aspects of the client's environment. A salient factors approach is client-focused care that addresses the long-term needs and goals of the client at the very beginning of the health care process to establish a treatment approach that effectively uses and manages resources. The salient factors approach

- Focuses on the key issues for each specific client, designing a plan that incorporates that client's involvement in care, streamlines care and captures care in a documentation format that reflects this process
- Focuses on the client's financial, human, and community resources from the onset of the injury or illness event, planning care within the bounds of those resources throughout the continuum experience
- Is outcome-oriented planning that assists in identifying barriers to discharge goals and outcomes, enhancing appropriate development of timely interventions

The salient factors approach drives the integration of the interdisciplinary process within a team. By asking "what are the five or six functions the client needs to be able to go home or to the next level of care?" the team's energy moves from the traditional establishment of "discipline goals" to a single list of *client goals* that reflects "that which the client needs," and results in client-driven care. Every team member is trained to reinforce (which is distinctly different from providing) all aspects of the client's plan of care, resulting in a 24-hour learning environment and accountability for outcomes by all staff members, regardless of discipline.

As complex and sophisticated information systems are being established in the care continuum, we must elevate their use from a purely financial and organizational foci to a communication and documentation system that will facilitate clinical care. Timely and consistent communication is the key to implementing the plan of care. The development and implementation of an interdisciplinary documentation system throughout the continuum supports every aspect of the process. When the initial client assessment is carried out by several team members at one time in partnership with the client, redundancy is virtually eliminated, and each team member hears and sees the same things. Everyone can focus on the key issues based on what the client needs, where the team is going, and what it will take to generate desired outcomes. Staff members can share their interpretations of observations and teach each other different aspects about the client from their areas of expertise.

Client-driven care planning that clearly defines the long-term discharge and short-term goals in measurable terms enables staff to know the parameters in which they are working and what is expected. In addition, when specific interventions are clearly outlined so every member of the team or family who comes in contact with that client uses the exact same technique each time, consistent ongoing training is provided to the client and the confusion about the "right" way is eliminated.

With every team member assuming equal accountability for outcomes, the continuance quality improvement (CQI) process can be elevated to a new standard of performance. Territories are eliminated and new awareness for staff capabilities opens. The interdisciplinary functional approach allows all team members to work consistently on the same goals for and with the client, contributing their unique expertise with the same techniques or methods each time. In addition, it helps the team coordinate the client's needs within the available time, resources, or limitations. For example, if a family needs to learn how to transfer a client before discharge, but family members are available only after 8:00 p.m. each evening, does that mean the physical therapist must be there or come back to teach them? In an interdisciplinary model the staff can assume that task, becoming accountable to the client and the rest of the team to reach that goal. Likewise, if a client is on a bladder training program and needs to void in the middle of a therapy treatment, the therapist can toilet the patient using therapeutic transfer and dressing techniques while reinforcing the patient's bladder training regimen. In this model, the legs and the transfer do not belong to the PT and bladder to the RN. They all belong to the client. The client and care time function as a unified whole to reach the desired outcomes.

It is important to note that *interdisciplinary does not mean* that the PT designs the bladder program and the RN designs the transfer protocol. An interdisciplinary environment means that each discipline specifically trained in certain aspects of care develops the client's care plan in that discipline's area of expertise and then collaborates and communicates it clearly to the team. In this way the program is enacted and reinforced to meet desired outcomes.

The true implementation of interdisciplinary team plans takes desire, time, facilitation, and constant reinforcement. The "upfront" investment at times seems overwhelming. The client outcomes, however, become incentives to the client, family, and staff, and the productivity and cost implications form the incentive structure for the health care facility and payor. The best part of this approach to a continuum of care strategy is that it is client focused and calls all team members to more creative, higher levels of practice.

FINAL THOUGHTS

We are moving from an illness-focused era to a wellness-focused era. This is an interim step in moving into the new paradigm that strives to potentiate the maximum fullness of life of a transglobal society. Moving to a democratic and compassionate society depends on equal access to information and shared decision making for all. This requires that every major organization and professional group ask broader, more inclusive questions. It demands a refocusing on issues that transcend personal interests to those of global dimensions. Enlarging our reality allows us to think and move in bigger circles, experiencing greater degrees of freedom and access to more resources and opportunities. We will leave an era of limitation and scarcity for an era of abundance.

Moving to that new reality is based on our understanding the connectedness of things. Kaiser (1995) identifies three things that must be integrated if transformation of this scale is to be achieved. Geographic mapping occurs as we identify the various resources available within our service area. Functional mapping defines what services are available within each of the agencies. Relational mapping assesses how well these arenas of service relate to each other. When the three are integrated to an inclusive whole, a new system is born. When customized to the unique needs and desires of the client, life-giving care is provided.

The rich and unique work of nursing has traditionally been at the bedside, one-on-one with the client. We will find work for some nurses in bedside caregiving roles in various service settings. What will be different is that some of them will provide physical care whereas others will provide discharge planning and education relating to health promotion or chronic illness lifestyle adjustment. We will also find some nurses in advanced practice roles facilitating and integrating care across the continuum of care. They will offer care that is complementary but different from the care available from primary care physicians as they focus on functional health status related to clinical pathology. As the definition of health is redefined to include social issues such as violence, poverty, and homelessness, we will find some nurses emerging in leadership positions at various corporate and legislative tables. Advocating for aggregate client populations rather than for a single patient, these nurses will lobby for social reform activities that can improve the health status of society.

Clearly, there is not a scarcity of health care issues or work to be done. It is equally clear that individuals in all disciplines who can see the larger reality of our complex society and modify past performance to appropriately meet these changing needs will have a critical place in the restructured health industry. If we simply reconnect with our roots, we will discover that Florence Nightingale called nursing to demonstrate a social conscience through the demonstration of social action with application of social imagination. If we heed her call, we will be a powerful force for health care reform.

REFERENCES

Burgess, C. S. (1995, November). *Information, opportunities, attitudes: Transitioning nurses to health care leadership. A fore for the future.* Speech given at the Association of Rehabilitation Nurses 21st Annual Education Conference, Indianapolis.

Burgess, C. S., & Balch, C. A. (1993). Rehabilitation nursing education and practice: Innovative responses to a changing delivery system. In C. J. Durgin, N. D. Schmidt, & L. J. Fryer (Eds.), *Staff development and clinical intervention in brain injury rehabilitation* (pp. 271-286). Baltimore, MD: Aspen.

Kaiser, L. (1995, June). *Transformational nursing leadership for the 21st century.* Speech given to the Leadership Institute for Nurse Executives at The Network for Health Care Management, Berkeley.

Melville, K. (1992, January). *Professions and professional relationships.* Speech given to Fielding Doctoral Students at Winter Session, Santa Barbara, CA.

Murphy, E. C. (1995). *Data-driven work redesign: Reducing operating costs and patient mortality while improving quality.* Amherst, NY: E. C. Murphy.

Small, J. (1992). *Transformers: The artists of self-creation.* Marina del Rey, CA: DeVorris.

CHAPTER 2

Ethical Issues for Nurse Administrators in a Changing Environment with Evolving Roles

Judith A. Erlen

The influence of evolving managed care forces on acute care hospitals and the vision of futurists and nurse leaders provide the backdrop for identifying and examining ethical issues that will challenge nurse administrators at the beginning of the 21st century. These ethical issues include, but are not limited to, the primacy of the patient, advocating quality care, acting in a just manner, challenging institutional policies and practices, and fostering organizational integrity. As managed care evolves, hospital nurse administrators will need to examine both new and reframed ethical questions. Seeking resolutions to these ethical dilemmas will challenge these nurse administrators to balance the goals of quality patient care and of the organization.

Generally speaking, the predictions of futurists are targeted at society at large; however, their projections also have implications specific to the evolution of the nursing profession in acute care hospitals. In *Megatrends,* John Naisbitt (1984) claimed that as society becomes more technologically driven there will be a corresponding need for a high touch counterpoint. He described a movement toward an information society in which knowledge is valued; the need for organizations to determine the focus of their business; and the already occurring population shifts. More recently, Naisbitt and Aburdene, in *Mega-trends 2000*, identified a trend that calls for a new respect for the individual and emphasizes the "primacy of the consumer" (1990, p. 307). Health care and nursing will be buffeted by these external forces and challenged to grapple with the ensuing ethical issues as nurses' roles evolve.

Nurse leaders have also looked to the future to identify ways in which the delivery of nursing care will need to change in light of health care trends. The use of technology is and will continue to be an integral part of nursing care, so nurses must examine how they view the caring component of nursing within a technologic environment and form an interface between technology and the individual patient (Aydelotte, 1988; Chinn, 1991). In addition, nurses will be involved in making decisions about how to allocate available resources in a just manner. As resources become scarcer, the demand for them will increase; life and health care decision making will become increasingly more complex (Chinn, 1991).

As the health care system changes, the patient's length of stay in a hospital is decreasing, more care is occurring in community and home-based settings, hospitals are downsizing their inpatient bed capacity, and the staff mix is changing with an increasing number of unlicensed personnel providing patient care (Cherbo, 1995). Costs are a major force driving the decisions of health care organizations. To contain costs, payers and administrators place controls over the services that are available. Containing costs is essential; however, this goal potentially can have a negative effect on the quality of patient care (Council on Ethical & Judicial Affairs, 1995). Thus, nurse administrators are challenged to make organizational decisions that do not sacrifice quality of patient care to control costs (Camunas, 1994a; Himali, 1995).

Because of the rapidity with which change is occurring in health care delivery, nurse administrators will need to anticipate what the future holds and be proactive rather than reactive decision makers. Finding appropriate resolutions to the ethical issues that the dramatic changes in health care are creating will require hospital-based nurse administrators to take risks and to consider new possibilities. Nurse administrators will need to be leaders, work cooperatively with members from other health disciplines, and creatively solve problems resulting from dramatic and chaotic changes. As nurse administrators work with other health professionals within a managed care environment, they must create a vision that is mindful of caring as the central moral value of nursing (Sullivan & Deane, 1994; Valentine, 1989).

The appearance and growth of managed care and the visions of futurists and nurse leaders provide the backdrop for the identification and exploration of new or reframed ethical issues that will challenge nurse administrators. The purpose of this chapter is to profile selected nursing ethical issues and discuss their parameters for nurse administrators under managed care imperatives. These ethical issues include, but are not limited to, the primacy of the patient, advocating quality care, acting in a just manner, challenging institutional policies and practices, and fostering organizational integrity. The challenge that each of these ethical issues brings will provide opportunities for nurse administrators to use creativity and skill.

Nurse administrators must recognize that their role has an ethical component (Camunas, 1994a). They must acquire the necessary knowledge, offer and use their expertise, and become actively involved in discussions and decisions related to ethical issues. In finding ways to resolve nursing ethical dilemmas, nurse administrators must keep the competing goals of quality patient care and of sound fiscal management within the organization balanced and in proper perspective. Nurse administrators will have a crucial role to play in demonstrating the significant difference that nursing can make in this changing health care environment.

PRIMACY OF THE PATIENT

The main reason that many individuals originally choose a career in nursing is to help others and to make a difference in their lives. Because nursing is a human enterprise, there is concern for the individual's health and well-being and a desire to provide ways for another to have an improved quality of life. The patient is of primary importance; nurses are human advocates (Curtin, 1979). The introduction of managed care has caused nursing to question nurses' traditional views of the patient and to reexamine both its reason for existing and the focus of its endeavors.

Managed care is creating changes within nursing and all of health care delivery. Nurses no longer approach patient care solely from the acute care hospital model of the bedside care nurse because of reengineered role opportunities and constraints being imposed by this new health care management system (Aiken & Salmon, 1994). For example, clinical care now can be expanded to incorporate complex care coordination to populations and groups of covered lives. Nursing responsibilities are shifting from particular patients to communities.

Nursing is a moral enterprise built on a foundation of trust (Erlen & Mellors, 1995). Nurses need to be true to the promise they make to society to care for patients, both individuals and aggregates. Nurses cannot merely follow organizational orders or yield to pressures from others in matters of patient care. Professional values and ideals have to guide their decisions. Nurse administrators and all nurses in the organization must be responsible and accountable for all of their actions. "Nurse administrators . . . must provide the necessary support and direction for caring to be evident within their practice environment" (Valentine, 1993, p. 329). Further, they have to play a vital role in challenging the health care system to higher moral decision making.

The "bottom line"—both quality outcomes and tight budgetary constraints —is a major concern in all health care organizations. When costs alone are the main focus, patients and their well-being cannot be the primary concern. This situation creates a conflict of interest for many nurse administrators. There is a "conflict between the economizing necessary for survival and growth and the presentation of behavior representing care and compassion" (Aydelotte, 1988, p. 8). Attention to methods of decreasing costs can compromise the interests of patients when services are arbitrarily reduced (Rodwin, 1995). One of these services is nursing care. Being labor-intensive, nursing care has been targeted for the most severe downsizing. Downsizing is affecting nursing's traditional role of bedside care provider and creating difficult ethical dilemmas for nurses.

One ethical dilemma facing nurse administrators centers on the competing interests of the patient versus those of the health care organization (McDaniel & Erlen, 1996). Nurse administrators are caught between these two interests because of their dual roles as nurses/patient advocates and as administrators. In a sense, nurse administrators wear two hats. The nurse administrator's role is to span the organization-patient interface and link the two together. Incorporated in this role are multiple obligations that can directly conflict with each other. Ordering these obligations can create major ethical conflicts. Nurse administrators need to ask themselves whether they can support the various goals of the organization. Does supporting these goals conflict with one's personal and professional values? Are the agendas of other members of the organization focused on maintaining quality within a cost-containment environment or is there some hidden agenda potentially creating ethical conflict for nurse administrators? Lehman (1994) warned nurse managers that "each day of your organizational life you will be challenged to perform in ways that could conflict with your natural tendencies" (p. 6). Creativity, innovation, and leadership can arise from the successful balancing of conflicting role demands and expectations, however.

Integrity is vital. For example, nurse administrators should not eliminate nursing positions in the organization just because they are told to do so; this action has the potential to jeopardize patient care. Nurse administrators must examine their professional values and determine whether such decisions are in accord with moral leadership, sound management, and organizational and personal professional values (Yeo & Ford, 1991). Then they must act with care and reason. Decisions have to be made because they are deemed to be ethically right and not because administrators are being pressured into particular decisions. As a result, acting with integrity for nurse administrators may mean that they take significant risks, that is, potential loss of job or potential decrease in decision-making responsibility, for themselves to support the goal of quality patient care. These personal risks can be offset, however, by the use of analyzed data, sound administration, and a strong moral compass to persuade and negotiate.

The mission of health care organizations and nursing should be to maintain or restore health or enable a peaceful death. This mission puts the needs of the patient/consumer first. Organizational decisions must intricately balance and coordinate the needs for patient care services and the attending costs so that the quality of patient care is not sacrificed.

ADVOCATING QUALITY CARE

Three examples of strategies that have been instituted to control the rising costs of health care include increasing the nurse-patient ratio, cross-training nurses, and increasing the number of unlicensed assistive personnel (UAP) who are hired and trained by health care organizations (Crawley, Marshall, & Till, 1993). Although these initiatives have the potential to decrease costs because fewer professional nurses may be necessary to provide care to a group of patients, there is also the strong potential that patients may be harmed and the care that is delivered may not be quality care (Aiken & Salmon, 1994; Himali, 1995). Clearly, care delivery systems must reconfigure if duplication and waste are to be avoided, yet this reconfiguration must ensure that patient outcomes do not suffer.

One of the two most significant responsibilities creating ethical dilemmas for nurse administrators is advocating for and monitoring the quality of care provided by professional nurses and by assistive nursing personnel within the organization. The other issue is managing scarce resources (Camunas, 1994a). Patients expect that they will receive quality care given by a competent staff of nurses at a reasonable cost. The expectation is that the appropriate nurse-patient ratio is available to deliver services that promote positive patient outcomes. "Beyond a critical ratio—that may be very difficult to determine with any precision—the quality of care will suffer" (Yeo & Donner, 1991, p. 163). Thus, personnel decisions that nurse administrators make must be in accord with the needs of both patients and professionals.

The ethical principle of nonmaleficence provides a basis for understanding and clarifying the issues related to providing due care and confronting unsafe practices. Nonmaleficence refers to refraining from engaging in harmful actions and not placing others at risk of harm (Beauchamp & Childress, 1994; Silva, 1990). Providing due care requires that one act in accord with defined standards so that there are good outcomes and a decreased burden for patients. The potential benefits of cost savings to the organization need to be balanced against the potential risks to patients as a result of the changes in the number and mix of staff. As their roles evolve, nurse administrators need to use ethical principles to examine both new and reframed ethical dilemmas.

Nurses know how to give appropriate traditional acute-care based patient care; however, some changes resulting from fiscal tightening mean that nurses have larger caseloads of patients and less time to spend with each one. If there is an insufficient number of nurses to care for patients and no other staff adjustments are made, nurses will have to work harder to provide patient care or accept an end result that most likely will not be high-quality care. When professional nurses are required to care for a larger number of patients, there is the increased likelihood of mistakes, such as medication errors, treatments not given, or patients and their families being neglected. Nurses will become tired, frustrated, and angry as they are asked to do more with less. The probability is that nurses will experience work-related stress and burnout and leave the occupation or organization. The result will be fewer nurses to care for the patients and the potential for increased errors, harm, and decreased quality of patient care.

Cross-training of nurses provides one possible resolution to the problem of uneven staffing patterns in the organization and a way to ensure that there is an adequate number of nurses on a given patient care unit of a hospital. Yet unless nurses can use these newly acquired skills or care for different types of patients, they will be unable to do so when the need arises. In addition, when staff are reassigned to another unit, they may not be familiar with the patients for whom they are caring. This situation creates an increased delegation/supervision workload for the unit nurses who now have the additional responsibility of helping to orient the staff who have been reassigned. Thus, the potential for human error increases if nurses are not as skillful in performing procedures and providing the care that their patients require. This issue surfaces again when hospital-based nurses are asked to cross-train for home health or long-term care settings.

Analogous to the population shifts occurring in the United States is the shift in health care to the strategy of an increasing use of UAPs as a way to provide less costly care. These individuals are nonprofessionals who are "trained to function in an assistive role to the licensed professional nurse in the provision of patient/client care activities as delegated by the nurse" (American Nurses

Association [ANA], 1993, p. 8). They are usually provided limited training by the organization that can view the use of UAPs as a "quick fix" to cost containment and staffing problems. Nurses' responsibilities are redistributed and UAPs are assigned to many of the patient care tasks (Erlen & Mellors, 1995; King, 1995). This change has created the need for nurses to delegate appropriate patient care activities to UAPs and to provide more direct supervision to UAPs (King, 1995). These responsibilities can draw professional nurses away from direct caregiving and absorb patient care time. Another problem occurs when UAPs merely replace RNs, because unlicensed individuals cannot provide the same level of patient care as professional nurses. UAPs lack the knowledge necessary to make complex clinical judgments about changes in patients' conditions. Therefore, appropriate professional intervention may be delayed, causing patients' well-being to be jeopardized.

The American Nurses Association (1993) developed a position statement to address the issue of the inappropriate use of UAPs within the varied health care settings. This position statement, along with a clear understanding of the state's nursing practice act and the *Code for Nurses* (ANA, 1985), can assist nurse administrators in advancing nursing's role and responsibilities related to the use of UAPs within the organization. To ensure that quality patient care is given, nurse administrators have to be intimately involved in developing policies about delegating nursing tasks to UAPs (King, 1995).

Because delegation of UAPs must be a nursing responsibility, nurses have to carefully assess the capabilities of UAPs before assigning any tasks. Many nurses lack the educational and experiential preparation in management and delegation skills, however. Therefore, without inservice education, they are unable to effectively assign patient care responsibilities and manage the available personnel resources, meaning that patients may be placed at risk. As advocates for quality care, nurse administrators must provide staff development programs on delegation and other management skills to minimize any risk to patients being cared for by UAPs.

ACTING IN A JUST MANNER

Many of the ethical concerns that are raised as a result of managed care forces focus on the patient-provider relationship (Council on Ethical & Judicial Affairs, 1995). Equally important, however, are the allocation decisions that must be made to adjust the number and composition of staff. Within any organization, there is a need to distribute the available services to patients. The ethical principle of justice provides a means for understanding concerns related to the availability and distribution of health care workers.

Managed care forces have created alterations in the delivery of health care services and related deployment of nursing services. Two changes affecting nursing staff are the expansion of hospital outpatient services and the reduction in the number of inpatient acute-care hospital beds (Cherbo, 1995). These changes reflect the shift in hospitalized patient populations. Fewer beds are needed when patients have shortened stays and can receive care in less costly ways. These changes suggest a different staff mix and different service utilization patterns. There may be an increase in UAPs. Other changes created by shortened hospital stays include more outpatient and home care, as well as the increased use of advanced practice nurses to provide health services.

Nurse administrators are being required to bring their budgets into line with these rapid changes. Generally, the only reactive ways to do this are by decreasing the size of the staff, controlling wages, and asking the remaining staff to work harder and smarter. Proactively, program strengthening and income generation strategies can be used. The ethical questions facing the nurse administrator include how to make personnel adjustments in a fair and equitable way and how to preserve the rights of nurses as employees when reengineering decisions are being made. Professional nurses expect that their nurse administrators will act in their staff's best interests and that administrators will act in accord with what is best for the organization, nursing, and patient care. Nurses, though, are beginning to question this commonly held perspective. Cuts and changes that are proposed and subsequently implemented in organizations are not being viewed as fair. Nurses see these institutional decisions as being made without a concern for the individual or as being discriminatory (Larkey, 1993). Staff may complain that the only concern is with the "bottom line"; there is no loyalty to or consideration for people and the contributions that they have made to the organization. Staff may be asked to work overtime or a double shift so that there is adequate coverage for the number of patients on the hospital's unit. Staff may ask, "If we are always being asked to work extra hours, why don't they hire more nurses?"

Ethical decision making balances bare-bones slashing of staff with justice in allocating scarce resources. Nurse administrators play a key role in insisting on distributive justice when making staffing decisions. Justice includes both the notion of fairness and what one is owed (Beauchamp & Childress, 1994; Rawls, 1971). Fairness suggests that decisions are made or individuals are treated so that there is no discrimination. For example, if the number and type of positions are constricting, affected nurses should be offered opportunities to reorient or reeducate themselves with the necessary new skills.

Principles of distributive justice can assist nurse administrators in making and justifying decisions regarding the redistribution of resources (Silva, 1990).

One guide to decision making is treating all equally. Do all nurses get an extra patient in their caseloads even if they have different abilities or different types of caseloads? A second principle is distributing according to need. Do some nurses get an increase in caseload and others have no change because some patients require more care? A third guide is to distribute according to ability. In this instance, some staff, because they have more expertise, may get the more challenging patients to care for while other nurses with less experience or ability may have fewer or less challenging patients in their caseload.

When allocating human resources using the principles of distributive justice, nurse administrators need to evaluate the situation carefully. The acuity or complexity of the situation and the available staff mix have to be considered. The ethical principle of nonmaleficence and the moral ideal of caring must also be considered. After weighing these various considerations, nurse administrators can then select any of the three identified ways of allocating resources as the ethical justification for their decisions.

The second perspective on distributive justice refers to giving to a person what the individual is owed and involves the notion of entitlement. Staff are entitled to be treated with respect. Although the organization does not owe a staff nurse a position, it does owe that individual due respect. Ways that nurse administrators can show respect include informing staff of organizational decisions in a timely manner and offering choices of alternative positions when possible.

As nurse administrators face issues of cost containment and cost reduction, tension is created because of the impact on the workforce. Staff can become disgruntled with the working conditions and the quality of care may suffer. Although nurse administrators are concerned with the larger systems perspective, they must also be concerned with the impact on the individual nurse and the ultimate affect on patient care. Nurse administrators must treat the nursing staff justly and with due respect. This means balancing and coordinating the needs of patients and staff with those of the organization.

CHALLENGING POLICIES AND PRACTICES

The traditional policies and practices that have served nursing and patients in the past have been or are being reformulated within the framework of managed care pressures. Managed care is creating a new way for nursing to be practiced. Clinical paths, one component of managed care, are being developed to ensure that patient care is coordinated and that patient outcomes are improved (Rudisill, Phillips, & Payne, 1994).

In developing these clinical paths, the nurse administrator should be an advocate for both patients and nurses. The administrator should strategically place nurses on institutional task forces that are creating clinical paths. In this way, the nursing perspective can become an integral part of all clinical pathways, and nursing can fulfill its role of being an advocate for patients.

Equally important to the development or adoption of these clinical paths is their evaluation (Schoenbaum, 1995). The only effective way to determine whether quality care is being delivered is to measure the outcomes and track the variances. Evaluation research is the means to determine whether clinical paths are doing what they are supposed to be doing and whether they are the most sound. If the outcomes are less than expected then the protocols need to be modified so that the goal of providing quality care can be achieved.

Using protocols such as clinical pathways can lead to coordination, efficiency, and standardization. The implementation of protocols requires that nurses make judgments about the benefits and risks to specific patients. What happens, however, if the patient's clinical course differs or does not fit the norm suggested by the protocol? Because the protocol will not serve the patient as well, the possibility exists that the patient can be placed at some risk. Therefore, ultimately such protocols have to be "implemented patient by patient" (Asch & Hershey, 1995, p. 850).

With the recent cuts in the number of nursing positions occurring within health care organizations, nurses may be reluctant to challenge policies that put patients at risk. Nurses may fear reprisals such as being ostracized, losing their jobs, or having work relationships change if they take positions that differ from those of the organization. Even nurse administrators may be hesitant to speak out because of these same fears. The *Code for Nurses*, however, requires nurses to challenge patient care practices whenever they put the patient at risk (ANA, 1985). Nurses must work to provide and maintain a patient care environment that fosters quality nursing care.

Nurse administrators also must be concerned with how proposed changes will affect the people who are responsible for actually making the change. Administrators have to consider the impact of change on the staff and on the organization. Will the changes strengthen or weaken the organization? Nurse administrators have an ethical responsibility to examine the effects of any planned change and to challenge those ideas that do not fit within a philosophy of caring or do not improve patient outcomes (ANA, 1985).

From a broader societal perspective, nurse administrators need to become politically active and address the evolving health care practices and policies. The nursing position needs to be stressed, particularly when so much emphasis is being placed on costs. Nurse administrators must become well-informed about the issues, develop their political skills, and gather the necessary data to support their position (Mason & Leavitt, 1995). In addition, nurse administrators can join with other nurses and support the campaigns promoting quality patient care initiated by the ANA, as well as the various state organizations. Through these means, nurse administrators will be able to influence evolving health care policies more effectively.

FOSTERING ORGANIZATIONAL INTEGRITY

Nurse administrators have to be concerned about both personal integrity and organizational integrity for the decisions that are being made. To foster organizational integrity requires that the values of the organization be clearly communicated (Paine, 1994).

The mission statement should express those values and ideals that the organization believes are important guides to the delivery of quality patient care. Their importance only becomes known, however, when administrators act in accordance with those values or take appropriate action when these ideals are violated. Are there strategies to facilitate a reflection on the values of the organization when decisions are being made? Decisions that are made need to reflect and incorporate the organizational values. Actions that result from these decisions also must reflect those values.

Because they span two constituencies, nurse administrators have to examine both their professional and the organization's values. As advocates for ethical practice, nurse administrators have to raise questions whenever those values conflict. Nurse administrators who are part of the decision-making body have an ethical responsibility to question any organizational decisions that do not fit with their professional ideals.

Nurses in administrative positions have a professional responsibility to create and foster an ethical environment within their organizations (Camunas, 1994a; McDaniel & Erlen, 1996). Such an environment will help instill ethical behavior among all levels of personnel. Nurse administrators need to ask questions and analyze the organization's policies and actions to ensure that there is an ethical environment. Are the values and ideals in the mission statement of the organization focused on patient care? Are decisions being made within this mission of the organization?

Likewise, nurse administrators have to empower the staff to make decisions that reflect the values of the nursing profession and foster organizational integrity. Systems have to be in place in the organization that recognize and support these ideals. Nurse administrators have to inspire loyalty and commitment to these values. Although there must be the expectation that these ideals support the practice of professional nursing within the organization and foster quality care, a caring environment that promotes the practice of nursing must also exist (Valentine, 1993).

Nurse administrators must provide a forum within the structure of the organization so that nurses have a mechanism to discuss ethical issues raised by the changes in health care delivery (Camunas, 1994b). Forums for discussing these ethical issues can provide nurses with the necessary skills to identify and analyze ethical dilemmas as they occur in their practice. Through the use of ethical analysis and reasoning, ethical dilemmas can become clearer, and ethically defensible resolutions can be determined. These forums will also enable nurses to get affirmation from other nurses that a proposed ethical action is justifiable. This supportive environment will then enable nurses to take the necessary moral actions.

Nurse administrators also need to hire nurse managers who understand and can communicate the values of both the organization and the nursing profession and who have the knowledge and the ability to make ethical decisions (Paine, 1994). Nurse managers, in turn, need to support their staffs in making ethical decisions. This way, nursing personnel within the organization can be expected to act in accord with a common set of values. These professional values are transmitted and reinforced, and all nurses become committed to them.

SUMMARY

Managed care, with its immediate focus on limiting hospital costs and services, challenges nurse administrators on two fronts: patient care issues and organizational issues. How can the patient's needs and quality care be kept primary in an environment in which the driving goal is to provide cost-effective and efficient service? How can nurses be enabled to have the freedom and opportunity to practice nursing as professionals and to be partners with other health professionals in providing patient care?

Providing quality care and not harming patients or placing them at risk has to be considered in relation to the benefits that patients have come to expect from nurses. Protecting the rights of nurses within this changing environment and allocating resources in a fair manner are other ethical concerns of nurse administrators.

As managed care evolves, nurse administrators will be called on to think about new or reframed ethical questions. In resolving ethical dilemmas, these administrators will have to consider the juxtaposition of the goals of quality patient care and the goals of the organization, balancing both for the sake of delivering high-quality and satisfactory patient care outcomes.

REFERENCES

Aiken, L. H., & Salmon, M. E. (1994). Health care workforce priorities: What nursing should do now. *Inquiry, 31,* 318-329.

American Nurses Association (1985). *Code for nurses with interpretive statements.* Kansas City, MO: ANA.

American Nurses Association (1993). Position statement on registered nurse utilization of unlicensed assistive personnel. *American Nurse, 25*(2), 8.

Asch, D. A., & Hershey, J. C. (1995). Why some health policies don't make sense at the bedside. *Annals of Internal Medicine, 122,* 846-850.

Aydelotte, M. K. (1988). The nurse executive in 2000 AD: Role and functions. In M. Johnson (Ed.), *Series on nursing administration, Volume I* (pp. 2-13). Menlo Park, CA: Addison-Wesley.

Beauchamp, T. L., & Childress, J. F. (1994). *Principles of biomedical ethics* (4th ed.). New York: Oxford University Press.

Camunas, C. (1994a). Ethical dilemmas of nurse executives. Part 1. *Journal of Nursing Administration, 24*(7/8), 45-51.

Camunas, C. (1994b). Ethical dilemmas of nurse executives. Part 2. *Journal of Nursing Administration, 24*(9), 19-23.

Cherbo, M. (1995, Spring/Summer). The shape of hospitals to come. *Advanced Practice Nurse,* 13-16.

Chinn, P. L. (1991). Looking into the crystal ball: Positioning ourselves for the year 2000. *Nursing Outlook, 39*(6), 251-256.

Council on Ethical and Judicial Affairs, American Medical Association (1995). Ethical issues in managed care. *Journal of the American Medical Association, 273*(4), 330-335.

Crawley, W. D., Marshall, R. S., & Till, A. H. (1993). Use of unlicensed assistive staff. *Orthopaedic Nursing, 12*(6), 47-53.

Curtin, L. L. (1979). The nurse as advocate: A philosophical foundation for nursing. *Advances in Nursing Science, 1*(3), 1-10.

Erlen, J. E. & Mellors, M. P. (1995). Managed care and the nurse's ethical obligations to patients. *Orthopaedic Nursing, 14*(6), 42-45.

Himali, U. (1995). Managed care: Does the promise meet the potential? *American Nurse, 27*(4), 1,14,16.

King, B. A. (1995). Working with a new staff mix. *RN, 56*(6), 40-41.

Larkey, L. (1993). Perceptions of discrimination during downsizing. *Management Communication Quarterly, 7*(2), 158-180.

Lehman, D. M. (1994). Manage from your ethics, not around them. *Seminars for Nurse Managers, 2*(1), 6.

Mason, D. J., & Leavitt, J. K. (1995). The revolution in health care: What's your readiness quotient? *American Journal of Nursing, 95*(6), 50-54.

McDaniel, C., & Erlen, J. A. (1996). Ethics and mental health service delivery under managed care. *Issues in Mental Health Nursing, 17*(1), 11-20.

Naisbitt, J. (1984). *Megatrends: Ten new directions transforming our lives.* New York: Warner Books.

Naisbitt, J., & Aburdene, P. (1990). *Megatrends 2000: Ten new directions for the 1990s.* New York: William Morrow.

Paine, L. (1994). Managing for organizational integrity. *Harvard Business Review, 72*(2), 106-117.

Rawls, J. (1971). *A theory of justice.* Cambridge, MA: Harvard University.

Rodwin, M. A. (1995). Conflicts in managed care. *New England Journal of Medicine, 332*(9), 604-607.

Rudisill, P., Phillips, M., & Payne, C. (1994). Clinical paths for cardiac surgery patients. *Journal of Nursing Care Quality, 8*(3), 27-33.

Schoenbaum, S. C. (1995). Health care reform and its implications for quality of care. *Medical Care, 33*(1, Supplement), JS37-JS40.

Silva, M. C. (1990). *Ethical decision making in nursing administration.* Norwalk, CT: Appleton & Lange.

Sullivan, J. L., & Deane, D. M. (1994). Caring: Reappropriating our tradition. *Nursing Forum, 29*(2), 5-9.

Valentine, K. (1989). Caring is more than kindness: Modeling its complexities. *Journal of Nursing Administration, 19*(11), 29-35.

Valentine, K. L. (1993). Utilization of research on caring: Development of a nurse compensation system. In D. A. Gaut (Ed.), *A global agenda for caring* (pp. 329-345). New York: National League for Nursing Press.

Yeo, M., & Donner, G. (1991). Justice. In M. Yeo (Ed.), *Concepts and cases in nursing ethics* (pp. 148-183). Lewiston, NY: Broadview.

Yeo, M., & Ford, A. (1991). Integrity. In M. Yeo (Ed.), *Concepts and cases in nursing ethics* (pp. 184-218). Lewiston, NY: Broadview.

CHAPTER 3

The Entrepreneurial Nurse: New Opportunities and Challenges

Richard W. Redman

Entrepreneurism presents exciting possibilities for nurses to deliver new services and products in today's health care marketplace. Establishing entrepreneurial ventures provides autonomy and flexibility for nurses in ways that generally do not exist within health care organizational structures. Setting up and running a business presents both opportunities and challenges for nurses in a rapidly changing competitive environment. This chapter examines entrepreneurship, its implications for nursing, and the risks and opportunities it offers.

The health care reform process that began in the early 1990s in the United States has stimulated a number of new roles and opportunities for many types of health care providers. One role that is seen with increasing frequency is that of nurse entrepreneur. Although nurses have always been involved in entrepreneurial activities, the extent and diversity of their entrepreneurial roles have increased dramatically as a result of the reformation process that is underway.

The rapid social and economic changes that seem to be endemic in the health care system provide ample opportunities and incentives to seek new ways of delivering services and meeting customer requirements. In society today, there is a strong demand for developing new technologies, new organizational structures, and new methods for service delivery across all kinds of industries. This is evident in health care as well. The emphases on health promotion and disease prevention, improved clinical outcomes, and quality service that is also cost-effective have provided opportunities that have not existed previously, especially for nursing.

The literature in nursing, with few exceptions, is silent on what entrepreneurs are, how to explore the options available, or how to become one. In addition, nursing education does not address entrepreneurism in any substantive way that might prepare individuals for undertaking new ventures. Although some guidelines and case studies are available in the literature, the entrepreneurial process appears more typically to be highly individualized and not shared with others. There are exceptions to this, but in general, nurses have to turn to the available general management literature on entrepreneurship and the strategies discussing how to become an entrepreneur.

This chapter examines the concept of entrepreneurship from a general business perspective as well as one specific to nursing. The term is defined and its relevance to nursing is discussed. Different types of entrepreneurial activities are examined with examples taken from the experiences of nurse entrepreneurs. The implications and challenges for potential nurse entrepreneurs in the rapidly changing health care environment are presented. Finally, implications for nurse administrators are presented.

ENTREPRENEURISM: WHAT IS IT?

The term *entrepreneur* originated from two French words, *entre* (between) and *prendre* (to take). The term was used in the Middle Ages to describe merchants who carried goods by ship or caravan between countries and across continents. It eventually came to mean "one who takes risks to gain profits," and this generally has been the most frequent interpretation. Today, the term entrepreneur seems to have a much broader meaning, describing someone who takes on a new business venture for a variety of personal reasons. The emphasis now is on new ventures and risk, rather than only profits.

We even have a variation on the role, that of *intrapreneur*, an intracorporate entrepreneur. This term describes individuals who take on new business ventures within an organization. It is now recognized that organizations need to have internal ventures so that they can flourish in today's marketplace. Intrapreneurs provide that leadership and innovation to help organizations compete effectively.

Vogel and Doleysh (1994) described a variety of elements conveyed in the term entrepreneur. Some aspects focus on the business perspective or operating one's own business; other aspects address innovation and creativity. With nursing in mind, they define entrepreneur as follows, "an individual who assumes the total responsibility and risk for discovering or creating unique opportunities to use personal talents, skills, and energy, and who employs a strategic planning process to transform that opportunity into a marketable service or product" (p. 4).

ENTREPRENEURSHIP: WHY NURSING?

The current environment, characterized by rapid social and economic changes, provides good reason as well as opportunities to seek new ways of doing business. In health care, there is a strong social and political emphasis on disease prevention and health promotion, developing technologies, vertical integration of health, and emphasis on clinical outcomes and quality. These are encouraging nurses to respond to opportunities that have not existed previously. Many of the health care services that are desired or demanded by consumers are those that can be provided best by nurses.

The variety of entrepreneurial opportunities available today also has relevance for nurses. Lonier (1994) pointed out that many women are seeing entrepreneurial ventures as a way to bypass the "glass ceilings" often faced in organizations. In addition, setting up one's own business provides independence that simply is not available in the corporate world. The organizational restructuring that often affects middle managers sometimes creates involuntary entrepreneurs. Individuals who are forced out of their positions often lose confidence in institutional approaches to problems. They feel that establishing their own ventures will give them opportunities that are not available within existing organizations. The motives for many entrepreneurs are more likely to focus on autonomy or a strong desire to shape their own careers around personal interests and lifestyles rather than fast growth and big monetary payoffs. Entrepreneurship is seen as the route to personal fulfillment.

Nursing products and services are often seen as value-added in today's fast-paced health care environment. As individuals and their families are forced to assume greater responsibility for caregiving, they find nurses an invaluable resource across the entire continuum of care. Consumers who desire primary care frequently turn to nurses who offer services that focus on health promotion, disease prevention, and risk reduction. Individualized plans of care that respect and value client preferences and needs are the hallmark of nursing practice. This, joined with cost-effective service at desirable levels of quality, places nursing in an enviable position in the marketplace.

ENTREPRENEURS: ARE THEY MADE OR BORN?

There is considerable interest in trying to determine what drives some individuals to become entrepreneurs. Studies have been conducted to identify the typical entrepreneur and develop a statistical prototype. Although some consistent traits are manifested by entrepreneurs, there does not seem to be an entrepreneurial "personality." Some individuals begin at a young age whereas others become entrepreneurs much later in life. Some individuals have a burning drive to run their own business, and others are forced into it. Entrepreneurs appear to be as diverse as any group of individuals.

Reports of research on qualities that successful entrepreneurs hold in common are available in the literature (Merrill and Sedgwick, 1993; Penderghast, 1994). Entrepreneurs consistently demonstrate a vision for creative or innovative ways of bringing a product or service to the marketplace. They are creative individuals who see possibilities for innovation and unique ways of doing something that generally are not apparent to others. They are industrious individuals who work very hard at whatever they undertake. Closely related to that, they work well independently and do not need a manager to ensure that they carry out their responsibilities. Stubbornness is another characteristic as evidenced by their thriving despite people who try to talk entrepreneurs out of their ideas. Resiliency is evident in their bouncing back readily from crises or setbacks. Finally, they are very responsible people who can deal with others—for example, employees in their business—counting on them to succeed.

Hosmer (1991) compared managers and entrepreneurs, finding they are not completely independent of one another. Managers can be contrasted with entrepreneurs, however, in that entrepreneurs tend to be more oriented toward future growth rather than current income and more inclined to use innovative rather than conservative methods. Hosmer described entrepreneurs as individuals who have high achievement needs. In addition, they have a tolerance of ambiguity, the ability to control events, and strong self-confidence. These qualities support the entrepreneur's ability to manage risk and uncertainty.

Vogel and Doleysh (1994) discussed gender differences between male and female entrepreneurs. In women, dissatisfaction with work experiences is often a major motivational force to forge out independently. Women are not searching for power or high income as much as the ability to achieve flexibility in balancing the multiple responsibilities they often face. Entrepreneurial activities provide freedom and flexibility which are frequently desired goals of women.

Gender differences also exist in management style and the type of companies that are established. Women frequently exercise power indirectly and are comfortable accomplishing goals through the efforts of others. Companies built by women have slower rates of growth, which is often advantageous in uncertain economic climates. Balancing multiple responsibilities is important to women and creating their own businesses fits with the many other responsibilities and roles women face. Women-owned companies tend to be smaller and are more frequently found in the service sector. The service sector offers both opportunities and threats; it presents lower barriers for developing a new company but also presents higher competition and greater difficulty in generating start-up capital (Vogel & Doleysh, 1994).

Some common characteristics are shown by entrepreneurs, but the results of the research are often contradictory. Overall, the conclusion is that the existence of single traits in an individual is not sufficient to predict either entrepreneurial behavior or success.

ENTREPRENEURIAL VENTURES AND NURSING

Merrill and Sedgwick (1993) have developed a useful typology for classifying entrepreneurial activities. They describe ventures that are idea-driven, idea-given, and idea-seeking. All three types have relevance for nursing.

Idea-driven ventures are those where the entrepreneur is the inventor. The idea can result in either a new product or service. The entrepreneur designs the product or service and then tries to sell it in the marketplace. This type of venture seems particularly relevant for nursing in today's rapidly changing health care industry. Several nurses have established businesses to deliver services that have been designed specifically to meet client and family needs in response to the dramatic decreases in acute care lengths of stay and the rapid shift to delivering health care services on an ambulatory or short stay basis. An example of this is nurses who have set up businesses to deliver lactation consultation services in the home to new mothers who are affected by shortened maternity stays in the hospital. Other examples can be found in nurse-run businesses that provide general nursing care or highly specialized services such as infusion therapy to clients in their homes.

A product example is the patient-assistive device designed and marketed by Dr. Clara Kimbro of Columbia, Maryland. She designed an inflatable pelvic lift device that makes it possible for one nurse or caregiver to single-handedly elevate a patient onto a bedpan or for other treatment purposes. The idea rose out of her several years of clinical practice and observing the difficulties in caring for immobile patients without endangering the safety of both caregivers and clients. She worked with design engineers, obtained a patent, and saw the product evolve from idea to market. Today she owns a company that designs products on the leading edge of caregiver technology (Kimbro, 1994).

The second category, *idea-given* ventures, are those that arise out of the entrepreneur's current position. The new business arises out of what the entrepreneurs-to-be do in their current positions. They see an opportunity to sell their expertise to others. This approach is very common with professionals who often act as consultants. A variation of this method that is becoming common in health care entails organizations selling their expertise and experiences to other organizations. For example, many hospital-based nursing departments that are very experienced with innovations, such as critical pathways or shared governance models, have set up revenue-generating ventures to provide consultations to hospitals interested in establishing similar programs.

The third category, *idea-seeking* ventures, entails entrepreneurs who search the current marketplace for opportunities, needs, or unmet demand. New ventures are then designed to produce a product or service to meet the potential demand. Leo Blatz, chief executive of Supplemental Health Care Services in Tonawanda, New York, provides a good example of a nurse entrepreneur who assessed the current market place for opportunities and unmet demand. He started a business in 1985 to meet the demands for supplemental nurse staffing. By 1994, he had built the business into a $10 million company placing nurses and physicians on four continents. The company was named to the *Inc. 500* list of fastest-growing companies in the United States (Blatz, 1994).

Nursing centers also illustrate this type of venture. Nursing centers are entities that provide clients direct access to nursing services and complete accountability and responsibility for client care remains with the professional nurse.

The first major study of nursing centers in the United States was conducted and reported by the National League for Nursing in 1993 (Barger & Rosenfeld, 1993). At that time, there were approximately 300 centers with the majority having been established since 1988. The majority of centers are affiliated with a parent organization, for example, a college of nursing or health care organization. The majority of centers provide primary care services including ambulatory care and health maintenance activities such as immunizations and screening. Newly established centers are more likely to care for vulnerable populations, such as homeless persons or HIV-infected individuals.

Another type of venture, not specifically addressed by the typology described, is the intrapreneurial venture or that undertaken by intracorporate entrepreneurs. Hollander and colleagues (1992) described a program at Stanford University Hospital that fosters risk taking among its nursing staff. This program has resulted in nurse-designed innovations such as the establishment of a short-stay surgical unit and a transitional care unit for stable geriatric patients and the development of cross-functional teams. Vogel and Doleysh

(1994) described the Hartford (Wisconsin) Memorial Hospital intrapreneurial program, which produced self-directed work teams in critical care units.

The typology and examples are not meant to be restrictive or inclusive. Rather, they are presented to illustrate the broad range of possibilities available to nurses. One might envision entrepreneurial ventures that cut across the categories described in various combinations. The types of entrepreneurial ventures possible in nursing are limited only by the ideas and visions of nurses themselves. Given the pro-entrepreneurial economy and the willingness of health care organizations to consider new ventures that might enhance their viability in the competitive market, the options available to nursing appear unlimited.

ISSUES AND RISKS FOR NURSING

Although the possibilities for nurse entrepreneurs have tremendous appeal, their new ventures are not without risk and challenge. Starting a new venture is extremely complicated and competition in the marketplace is fierce. Preparing to be an entrepreneur can also be quite challenging because most educational programs, including those in colleges of nursing and schools of business administration, do not prepare individuals with the kinds of skills needed for setting up a new business. Finally, the availability of capital for start-up ventures in health care is very limited because of the volatility and uncertainty in the industry. This section addresses each of these issues and their implications for nurse entrepreneurs.

Lonier (1994) reported that 8 out of 10 new businesses fail within the first three years of operation. The competition is severe and the risks are great. Obviously, having a good business idea is not sufficient to succeed. The odds are much better for businesses with one owner compared with those having multiple owners. Nearly 75% of solo-owned businesses are still operational after five years. This has relevance for nurse and women entrepreneurs. Vogel and Doleysh (1994) reported that nurse-owned enterprises tend to start out smaller and grow at a slower rate. These facts are no doubt related to the probability of long-term survival in the marketplace.

Some personal characteristics of entrepreneurs may contribute to the high rate of failure in their business ventures. Stancill (1981) pointed out that new ventures are at greatest risk of failing during their early years. The most important preventive action is for the entrepreneur to be "hard-nosed" in evaluating the ideas for the venture. Given their self-confidence, independence, and tolerance of ambiguity, entrepreneurs may move their idea into the marketplace prematurely without fully evaluating all aspects of the venture.

Market research strategies provide critical insights to the potential success for new products and services. Merrill and Sedgwick (1993) described "top-down" and "ground-up" market assessment techniques. In the top-down approach, the entrepreneur establishes that there is a potential market through reports produced by market research firms, industry projections typically found in trade magazines, and analyses of census statistics for market and consumer characteristics. A useful source of market information is a publication called *Predicasts*, which provides annual summaries of market research studies, indexed by industry. This is generally available in business school libraries. "Ground-up" market research entails generating sales projections through interviews with prospective purchasers of the new product or service. Another approach consists of surveying random samples of residents or businesses in the marketplace to identify potential customers, their purchasing preferences, and their assessment of competitor products and services in the market.

Veit (1992) stated that it is essential for the entrepreneur to identify with the customer, either potential or real. The entrepreneur must learn what the customer wants and then be sure it is delivered. Nurses should be well positioned for this because of their fundamental approach to clients as co-equals in determining plans of care. Translating this approach into identifying with the customer is likely to be a natural approach taken by the nurse entrepreneurs and could contribute to their success.

Learning how to set up a business venture is not a readily available educational process. Setting up a new venture is extremely complicated. The new entrepreneur needs a broad range of knowledge and skills or access to individuals with expertise in legal requirements, marketing, financial management and accounting, capitalization, liability issues, general management, reimbursement, and protecting the innovation, just to name a few. The general business literature offers a variety of strategies and recommended approaches, but in the end these are no guarantees of success. Hosmer and Guiles (1985) described the process of forming a venture by using a standard business plan development approach. Vogel and Doleysh (1994) recommended a variety of similar strategies to be followed. They also listed a variety of resources for nurses who want to establish their own businesses. Although these recommended approaches appear to be systematic and straightforward, case studies of entrepreneurial start-ups often present a different view. Vet (1992) aptly described the travails of establishing one's own business. Hard work and potential opportunities do not always produce success. External market factors can easily overcome personal capabilities, proven concepts, and solid capitalization.

The frequent lack of evaluation of the impact of entrepreneurial ventures also detracts from important learning opportunities that could guide those who might learn from the successes and failures of other entrepreneurs. Gray (1993) reviewed the literature covering nearly 20 years of experience with academic nursing centers. He found virtually no studies that evaluated the impact of nursing centers on the health outcomes of the clientele. It is essential that the impact of nursing ventures be evaluated by the outcomes they achieve, the products and services they produce, and the costs incurred. Impact evaluations would contribute important learning opportunities for all nurses who are thinking of designing ventures in the future.

The final challenge deals with the need for capital to fund the development and implementation of new ventures. Lonier (1994) discussed the most common methods used to finance new ventures. Self-funding is the major source of capital. This includes the use of personal savings or pooling money with colleagues and friends who will either join the new business venture or provide loans. Many entrepreneurs begin their ventures on a part-time basis while they continue to work full-time elsewhere. Loans from commercial banks are frequently used. The U.S. Small Business Administration (SBA) works with commercial banks to support small business development through guaranteed loans. The SBA is particularly interested in supporting new ventures headed by females or minorities. Venture capital, or funds from individuals or firms that invest in businesses for a profit, is often used if large amounts of capital are needed. Another source of funding that is becoming increasingly popular is working independently for a former employer who in turn becomes the first major client.

Tong (1995) described the constraints in the health care delivery system concerning the availability of capital to fund new ventures. Capitalization requires that decisions made must be selective and relevant to emerging models of delivering health care. Capital allocation in the future will be based on those ventures that will yield the highest return, not just conventional profit returns. Patient outcomes and their effect on the community will be central to evaluating what ventures are funded. Clearly, the contemporary availability of capital in the health care industry will be a major force for nurses to consider when seeking out ways to fund new ventures.

Nurse entrepreneurs need not be limited to capital sources that are available only in the health care industry. Vogel and Doleysh (1994), in their survey of nurse entrepreneurs, reported that 42 of the 50 respondents relied to some extent on personal funds to begin their businesses. About 60% of the nurse entrepreneurs started their businesses with less than $2,000. Although it appears that nurse-owned businesses can be established with a variety of sources of start-up funds, capital from health care organizations is likely to be increasingly difficult to acquire.

IMPLICATIONS FOR NURSING

The new opportunities, risks, and challenges that nurse entrepreneurs face have several implications for nursing. These include implications for nurse administrators, educators, and entrepreneurs themselves. All require bold action and breaking ingrained modes of behavior. Changing roles and ways of thinking may be threatening but also can produce growth and professional development.

As health care organizations struggle with the challenges they face in the marketplace, it appears that nurse entrepreneurial and intrapreneurial roles provide viable options for nurse administrators to use in designing and delivering new health care services and perhaps increasing market share as well. Nurse administrators can create the kind of organizational culture and climate that will foster innovations and new ventures. The nurse administrator is a key decision maker in allocating resources to support and encourage the development of the kinds of creative nursing entrepreneurial ventures that are beginning to develop. Clearly, making venture capital available would be an important catalyst for success. The incubator approach, used by many industries to nurture creative ideas and convert them into new products and services, is another approach that the nurse administrator could implement. Nurse administrators also have the responsibility to ensure that new entrepreneurial ventures are fully evaluated so that their affect is measured and the results are shared in the literature. This will permit others to learn from the successes and failures, and all will benefit in the end.

Nurse educators have a major responsibility in fostering and supporting entrepreneurship. Certainly, educators can be entrepreneurs themselves and they also can lead efforts within their colleges to design and implement new ventures. More important, educators need to ensure that students become familiar with entrepreneurial roles as an important career option in nursing. Incorporating concepts about entrepreneurship into the undergraduate and graduate curricula would provide important learning opportunities for present and future nurses. Collaborative efforts with other academic units, such as business schools, would also increase educational opportunities for nurses who want to acquire the knowledge base and skills for entrepreneurial roles. For example, academic nursing centers provide a rich opportunity for risk and adventure.

Finally, nurse entrepreneurs themselves have an important responsibility to share their experiences with the nursing community. Publications, seminars, and case studies that discuss the experiences that nurse entrepreneurs have had in establishing and running business ventures will make an invaluable contribution to present and future generations of nurses. Celebration of success stories communicates a positive image of the profession of nursing.

The challenges to becoming a nurse entrepreneur are both exciting and formidable. Clearly, the opportunities available to nurses who want to lead efforts that will bring new products and services to patients and their families have never been better. With the steadfast commitment that nurses have to providing cost effective patient centered services, entrepreneurial roles offer a critically important way for nurses to make substantial contributions to ongoing health care reform.

REFERENCES

Barger, S., & Rosenfeld, P. (1993). Models in community health care: Findings from a national study of community nursing centers. *Nursing & Health Care, 14,* 426-431.

Blatz, L. R. (1994). Personal communication.

Gray, P.A. (1993). Can nursing centers provide health care? *Nursing & Health Care, 14,* 414-418.

Hollander, S. F., Allen, K. E., & Mechanic, J. (1992, January-February). The intrapreneurial nursing department: Nature and nurture. *Nursing Economic$, 10,* 5-14.

Hosmer, L. T. (1991). *Entrepreneurial management: A guide.* Unpublished coursepack. University of Michigan School of Business.

Hosmer, L. T., & Guiles, R. B. (1985). *Creating a successful business plan for new ventures.* New York: McGraw-Hill.

Kimbro, C. (1994, May). *Entrepreneurial ventures for nursing: Development of a product.* Presentation made at the University of Michigan School of Nursing, Visiting Committee Meeting.

Lonier, T. (1994). *Working solo: The real guide to freedom & financial success with your own business.* New York: Portico.

Merrill, R. E., & Sedgwick, H. D. (1993). *The new venture handbook.* New York: Amacom, American Management Association.

Penderghast, T. F. (1994). Types of entrepreneurs. *Management & Organization Development 17,* 25-26.

Stancill, J. M. (1981, November-December). Realistic criteria for judging new ventures. *Harvard Business Review.* Reprint No. 81613.

Tong, D. (1995, June). Being good neighbors. *Hospitals & health networks 69,* 40-42.

Veit, K. (1992, November-December). The reluctant entrepreneur. *Harvard Business Review.* Reprint No. 92609.

Vogel, G., & Doleysh, N. (1994). *Entrepreneuring: A nurse's guide to starting a business* (2nd ed.). New York: National League for Nursing Press.

CHAPTER 4

Nurses as Policy Analysts and Advocates: Avoiding Lessons Already Learned

Lelia B. Helms
Mary Ann Anderson

The policy literature is rich with descriptions of lessons learned, usually the hard way. This chapter reviews the basic literature on the policy process and points to its potential utility for nurses interested in securing and enhancing the role of nursing in the changing health care delivery system. The motivation for this effort stems from a concern over the failure of nursing to date to draw on this literature when developing policy. To avoid the pitfalls of the policy process, nursing needs to capitalize on knowledge already available. A thorough understanding of the processes and environment of policy can assist nurses in articulating and sustaining a substantive, as opposed to symbolic, role in the health policy arena.

Over the past decade, policy has emerged as a cottage industry in many fields. With growing frequency, nurses have added their voices and claimed roles for themselves as policy analysts and advocates (Harrington & Estes, 1994; Lescavage, 1995; Mason & Talbott, 1985; Mason, Talbott & Leavitt, 1993). Typical of claims by nurses is the statement by Mitchell, Krueger, and Moody (1990): "The new public debate on health care reform gives nurses an opportunity to transform this ineffective market-oriented medical model into a universal, true health care system" (p. 214). Although participation by nurses in health policy making is necessary, an improved understanding by nurses of the processes that shape policy development is prerequisite to greater effectiveness in this area.

In the nursing literature on policy, there is limited evidence concerning how policy processes constrain the substance of health policy generally, and nursing policy specifically (Hanley, 1993; Sochalski, 1993). Without knowledge of the fit between the environment, process, and substance of policy, nurses interested in defining and influencing policy risk irrelevancy and marginalization. Good intentions and good ideas do not offset ineffectiveness attributable to a lack of understanding of policy processes.

The literature on policy processes and environment, gained from a wide range of fields employing policy-based perspectives, is useful to the general nursing community. It can contribute to development of a framework for refining nurses' roles as policy analysts, advocates, and administrators. In addition, this review of the broader nonnursing literature on policy processes is designed to broaden discussion about methods of advancing the policy interests of nursing.

POLICY BASICS

Policy is defined as "a purposive course of action followed by an actor or set of actors in dealing with a problem or matter of concern" (Anderson, 1975, p. 3). Policy reflects the application of reason and evidence to problem-solving, whether in public or private settings. The analysis of policy extends the approach of the scientific method to understanding how to transform substantive knowledge pertinent to human needs into delivery systems to serve those needs. Policy connects basic scientific knowledge to practice through a series of linkages, reliant on institutions, people, and processes.

Although policy relies on evidence generated by research and the scientific method as the substantive core of knowledge, understanding what happens to that knowledge as it is transformed into policy through a range of institutional processes requires discarding the dominant rational-linear problem-solving model as a common framework for understanding. The rational-linear paradigm depends on identifying and ordering objectives, comparing alternatives according to set criteria, and selecting the highest ranking as the goal of policy. In practice, however, understanding policy requires considering multiple factors including timing, resources, social and organizational interaction, preferences, politics, culture, and luck. The how and why of what policy choices emerge from the policy process defy simple explanation or ready prediction.

The rational paradigm cannot explain the relationship between policy knowledge and practice.

Policy analysis can be characterized as an activity that creates problems for which solutions are available (Kingdon, 1984). The identification of solutions, that is, strategies relying on readily controllable variables and resources, precedes and shapes how problems are defined. The availability of solutions, whether partial or comprehensive, is a necessary precondition for the problem definition and then for policy movement. Change depends on the evolution of solutions that are attached to, and subsequently redefine, problems. Indeed, "it could be argued that most problems are solved by redefinition, substituting a puzzle that can be solved for a problem that cannot" (Wildavsky, 1979, p. 57). Both policy solutions and problems are defined temporally as answers or limited successive approaches to endemic conditions or underlying needs (Schon & Rein, 1995). The major task for policy analysts is to "create problems that decision makers are able to handle with the variables under their control and in the time available" (Wildavsky, 1979, pp. 14-15).

Policy environment conditions relationships between policy problems and outcomes. Here, the analogy of space is useful, particularly when viewed ecologically. The newer and emptier a space is, the fewer the interactions between objects occupying that space, and the simpler the problems of developing and implementing policy without accommodation to other policies. As the number of programs addressing one policy sector increases over time, policy space becomes crowded. The reciprocal and interactive effects of change multiply, often with unintended or unforeseen consequences.

> Early occupants of a policy space are fortunate . . . newcomers will be forced to adjust to . . . existing programs . . . . No reduction of benefits (the usual "hold harmless" provision) is allowed for older programs; hence, benefits may actually increase for all . . . every time newcomers do better. (Wildavsky, 1979, p. 66)

These characteristics have both program and organizational implications. As policies are adopted and implemented, policies become programs, each with its own organizational framework delivering services or benefits to a constituency. Both territorial and functional differentiation produce disaggregated decision-making and delivery systems. The result is a multiplicity of policies that can be viewed as a collection of subsystems with limited tasks, competencies, goals, and resources. In crowded policy spaces, problem-solving capacity becomes ever more dependent on coordination and cooperation with other groups, organizations, or subdivisions (see Figure 4.1).

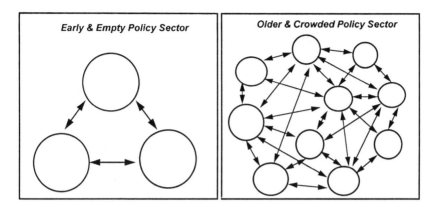

Figure 4.1: Policy Space

Similarly, in crowded policy spaces, the consequences of change become more unpredictable as the number of potential effects on other programs multiplies. Furthermore, other actors in the same policy space recognize the potential consequences of change on their program areas and incentives to mitigate such effects multiply. The result is often a trade-off, a deliberate decrease in any proposed policy change to minimize opposition, to enhance chances of adoption, and to decrease the number of spillover effects. Changes become incremental by design, limited in scope and consequence, because of their environmental impact rather than for any substantive merit. "As policy effects accumulate and interact, the explosion of costs becomes less important than the implosion of spillovers" (Heclo, 1975, p. 412). Over time, the possibilities as well as the forms of change become ever more constrained. The crowded health policy sector provides ample evidence of the effects of complexity on change.

In summary, policy involves the translation and application of knowledge to practice. Linking that transformation are processes and environments that shape and constrain outcomes. Policy is not isolated and abstract. Although the knowledge base that informs each policy sector may be distinctive, the processes by which it is translated into practice are not.

POLICY PROCESSES

Policy making is traditionally described as a five-stage discrete, linear, and progressive process (Anderson, 1975), as shown in Figure 4.2.

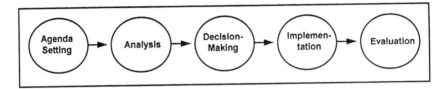

Figure 4.2: Policy Process

This model is useful for understanding the basic stages of policy making. As with most simplifications, however, it can also be misleading. In reality, policy making occurs in a dynamic, interactive environment with limited direction- ality and formality. The utility of the model of policy making that frames the remainder of this discussion must be understood within these limitations.

Agenda setting

The first stage in policy making is understanding how issues are identified for public consideration. The range of human problems is almost limitless. Time and attention are relatively scarce, however. Only a few problems can be addressed by the formal political process at any one time. There are always more problems and needs than time and resources to deal with them. The study of agenda setting seeks to understand how and why some issues and alternatives receive attention whereas others do not. Agenda setting examines the process by which perceptions of social needs are defined, aggregated, and formalized in public and governmental decision-making settings.

Kingdon's attempt to describe "what makes an idea's time come" in the two public policy areas of health and transportation over a period of three decades focused attention on the study of agenda setting (Kingdon, 1984, p. 1). Relying on Cohen, March, and Olsen's (1972) "garbage can model" of organizational decision making, Kingdon described agenda setting as the coupling of three streams: (1) problem recognition by the environment, (2) the availability of solutions, and (3) formal and informal political structures. The first stream, problem recognition, identifies mechanisms through which attention becomes fixed on one problem rather than another. These include indicators or data gathering mechanisms, crises, focusing events, and budgets. The second stream, availability of solutions, describes what Kingdon terms a "policy soup." The policy soup is composed of ideas and approaches in varying combinations, which are generated primarily by participants and experts within a specific policy sector and which, through a long developmental process of brokering and assessment, are refined into alternatives or proposed solutions. The third stream, the formal and informal processes of public decision making, contains the structural and opportunistic decision points available to politicians and policymakers for attaching solutions to problems and translating proposals into policies.

The coupling of these three streams produces windows of opportunity for policy entrepreneurs. Windows of opportunity for policy making are driven by events, which are relatively unpredictable, and by governmental and political processes, which are cyclical. Entrepreneurs are "people willing to invest their resources in return for future policies they favor" (Kingdon, 1984, p. 214). Policy entrepreneurs, defined as advocates or activists interested in policy change, play a "major part in the coupling at the open policy window, attaching solutions to problems, overcoming the constraints by redrafting proposals, and taking advantage of politically propitious events" (Kingdon, 1984, p. 174). Policy develops opportunistically in response to the shifting dynamics of events, actors, solutions, and problems.

Baumgartner and Jones (1993) extended and sharpened the analytic framework for understanding agenda setting and placed it within the interaction of various other stages in the policy process. They posit a theory of "punctuated equilibrium" to explain the emergence and decline of policy issues from the public agenda (p. 21). Supported by extensive case study data, they argued that policy undergoes long periods of stability and limited incremental change that are only rarely interrupted by very substantial, even radical, bursts of activity and reform.

When policy problems are initially addressed and programs developed, organizational structures are created that remain in place for decades. These structures shape participation, limit change, and preserve monopolies. They create the illusion of rigidity and equilibrium within a policy sector. Activists stifled by these equilibria, however, seek alternative outlets to voice their dissatisfaction and seek change. This occurs in two ways: by mobilizing the media and by changing the venue of political action. The federal structure of the American governance, by offering multiple forums for alternative approaches, is conducive to strategies of problem disaggregation and decentralization. Over time, dissatisfaction with existing policy builds. Those excluded from existing major policy subsystems constitute "slack resources" available for experimentation and generation of alternatives in the new and experimental venues, particularly at the state and local levels. Gradually, mobilized by policy entrepreneurs, momentum for change builds. Periodically, the energy generated by these building processes spills over into the national forum with dramatic force. The problem then is addressed, often radically, as a result of the scope of reform and prior experience. Baumgartner and Jones (1993) termed this characteristic of policy change, "punctuated equilibrium" (p. 21). Policy is characterized both by long periods of organizational stability and incremental policy making and by occasional, rapid, and radical shifts in policy approaches. Both are generated by the same underlying process.

The evidence from the 1993 to 1994 round of attempted health care reform illustrates the interaction of factors described in the agenda setting literature. Preceded by a long period of stability and incremental reform, and by a range of reform efforts in numerous but disparate venues, health care reform moved to the top of the national policy agenda briefly. A window of opportunity opened and then closed after exhausting its momentum and political resources for the time being. In part, a solution was not available to be attached to the problem in a timely enough manner to take advantage of the brief opportunity. Comprehensive policy change may be foreclosed in the health policy sector over the short term as actors and resources regroup. Health sector policy change, nonetheless, continues to occur, although in incremental and tentative localized steps, rather than in a nationally coordinated approach.

Analysis

The second stage in policy making involves the formulation of alternatives or proposals responsive to policy issues. The focus in this phase is on specifying alternatives and predicting consequences in terms of a range of policy options. The concern at this phase is "with how the decision maker should structure his thinking about a policy choice and with the analytic models that will aid understanding and prediction" (Stokey & Zeckhauser, 1978, p. 4). Policy analysis involves defining a problem, identifying the criteria by which the policy will be judged, and finally specifying a range of feasible approaches generated by applying predictive models to alternatives. "The criterion for good policy is not only what is 'right' but also what is a product of thorough analysis and what is feasible in the policy arena" (Rains & Hahn, 1995, p. 72).

The rational paradigm dominates thinking about substantive policy issues at this stage. The rational paradigm may be characterized by the following:

- Clarification of values or objectives is distinct from and usually prerequisite to empirical analysis of alternative policies.

- Policy formulation is therefore approached through means-end analysis: First, the ends are isolated, then the means to achieve them are sought.

- The test of "good" policy is that it can be shown to be the most appropriate means to desired ends.

- Analysis is comprehensive; every important, relevant factor is taken into account.

- Theory is often heavily relied on. (Lindblom, 1979, p. 81)

This paradigm served as the starting point for the development of interest in policy studies. It now constitutes the core of most academic programs in policy studies as well as in applied policy fields. This focus reflects the effort to reconcile and apply knowledge and research in systematic ways to practical social problems. In nursing to date, the rational paradigm constitutes the only lens through which policy is understood (O'Neill & Pedersen, 1992; Rains & Hahn, 1995; Stimpson & Hanley, 1991).

In the analysis stage, the focus is technical. Analysis often requires mastery of a variety of analytic models such as cost-benefit analysis, simulations, queuing techniques, decision analysis, linear programming, discounting, defining preferences, Markov chains, and difference equations (Stokey & Zeckhauser, 1978). Undergirding each are specific assumptions about behavior. This approach is premised on the idea that improved analysis results in better policy options and improved outcomes. As a consequence, policy studies usually concentrate on designing better substantive policy options, termed *models of choice*, which can produce results with greater generalizability and longevity to guide specific recommendations or solutions (Lindblom, 1991; MacRae & Wilde, 1985).

The utility of formal analytic policy approaches in practice settings may be limited (Schon & Rein, 1995). Knowledge is not institution bound. Policy decisions, however, are translated into programs embedded in organizations responsible for delivering services or products. A perennial, if not insurmountable, problem for analysts is how to reconcile knowledge with practice. Knowledge depends on learning and analysis, activities that identify errors and promote change. Organizations, on the other hand, depend on stability and replication of activities as criteria of efficiency and effectiveness. The primary function of information for organizations is to sustain core agency needs, functions, and resources (Wilensky, 1967). New information and knowledge have limited utility for organizations that have few incentives for restructuring or change. Despite the popular literature, particularly in public sector agencies, organizational learning is slow and episodic.

A similar conclusion characterizes findings about the utility of research to policymakers (Weiss, 1980). Policymakers tend to filter research through two screens: truth, or trustworthiness, and utility. Policymakers can identify research that is not relevant, of high quality, and nonconforming to organizational assumptions but report limited reliance on research as the basis for designing policy. As Weiss (1980) concluded,

A major reinterpretation that emerges . . . is the meaning of the "use of research." The conventional interpretation is the direct application of the findings of a study to the solution of a problem: A decision is pending, research provides information that is lacking, and with the information in hand, the decision maker makes a decision. Such uses occur, but they are rare. Particularly, when research is done outside the agency, the likelihood is small that a study's results will match the problems, information gaps and available options confronting a decision maker with sufficient exactness to be translated directly into action. (p. 263)

The study of health policy, generally, and nursing, specifically, is dominated by a focus on the substantive rationality of specific approaches to the detriment of understanding the processes of policy making, both at the decision-making and implementation stages. Indeed, the former is viewed as appropriate and useful, whereas the latter is viewed as belonging to the rather distasteful world of politics and politicians. There has been little integration or merger of the two as necessary and inseparable when designing policy solutions that have greater applicability to the organizational settings of nursing practice.

Decision Making

The decision-making stage relies on the formal processes of policy adoption. A policy choice is made through the procedures specified by organizational and public structures for governance. The number of possible policy options is narrowed to one and formally legitimized. In organizations, the degree of formality and structure in decision making can vary widely depending on agency culture and environment, as well as the scope of the problem. In the public arena, decision making involves the study of politics, particularly those political processes surrounding legislatures and the dynamics of legislation.

The study of public decision making is both structural and situational. It is structural in that legislatures employ formal, publicized, predictable, and accessible processes for making substantive policy decisions. It is situational because the dynamics of each case are created by the particular mix of specific issues, players, solutions, and timing—all of which interact idiosyncratically (Kingdon, 1984). Knowledge about decision-making structures and processes is widely available and accessible. Knowledge about decision making as applied to specific policy examples is more limited and reliant on the availability of case studies. In nursing, knowledge about structures for public decision making is becoming more readily available (Kalisch & Kalisch, 1982; Mason & Talbott, 1985; Mason, Talbott, & Leavitt, 1993). There are, however, fewer sophisticated case studies of substantive policy development and adoption in nursing, a gap that may have inhibited learning and limited the effectiveness of nurses' roles as participants in shaping health policy.

Finally, the processes of decision making are often misunderstood or misleading when decision making is viewed from the rational paradigm alone

(Allison, 1971). Most case study literature reviews policy decisions, which are then evaluated by comparison with some "best" option. Inevitable discrepancies between "ideal" policy options and actual policy choices are then attributed to the unscrupulous and irrational requisites of politics and power, compromise and bargaining, rather than the structural and procedural complexities of the policy and decision-making processes. Policy "rationality seems better understood as a postdecision rather than a predecision occurrence" (Weick, 1969, p. 38). Few policy decisions introduce sweeping, rational, or comprehensive change. Requisites of system stability and maintenance dominate policy decisions most of the time.

A more useful model for understanding policy outcomes and decision making views the process of making policy choices as biased toward incremental rather than comprehensive and rational policy change. Incremental policy choices reflect a better fit with decision-making structures in the public sector. American political institutions are decentralized and deliberately designed to slow decision making and to limit its scope (Madison, 1787-1788). Both the organizational principles of federalism and separation of powers reinforce this bias in American governance.

Incremental problem-solving is characterized by

- Choices made at the margins of the status quo
- Consideration of a limited number of policy alternatives
- Smaller rather than large changes
- Adjustment of policy goals to available means
- Adaptation of policy to changing circumstances
- Policy focused on correcting negatively perceived problems rather than on attaining goals (Braybrooke & Lindblom, 1963, pp. 81-110)

Incremental policy making depends on the interactive effects of multiple players in the policy process for ongoing feedback. Governance structures permit stakeholders to participate and to exert influence at many points. This requires the accommodation of interests among partisans. The results reflect the logic of compromise and mutual adjustment of interests rather than any consistent logic or rationality of policy. "In a participatory approach to governance it is much easier to prevent major change than to negotiate it" (Helms, 1981, p. 5). Change, when it occurs, is at the margin rather than at the center of policy. Over time, however, incremental approaches do result in substantial policy movement. Years of piecemeal changes to Medicare provide an example of the potential for substantial expansion in scope and substance resulting from such decision-making processes.

Implementation

Implementation is the stage in which policy decisions are translated into practice, that is, "getting the job done" (Jones, 1984, p. 165). Policy decisions provide a basic, broad outline or framework of goals and approaches to be filled in by agencies assigned responsibility for actual implementation. The process of implementation by which organizations transform policy decisions into practice is analogous to a series of wooden boxes nested one inside another as choices are made and responsibilities allocated with increasing specificity from the highest levels of administrative responsibility to staff on to practitioners delivering services in the field.

Interest in the study of policy implementation was stimulated by observations about persistent discrepancies between policy decisions, objectives, and outcomes and by efforts to address the "lack of fit" (Pressman & Wildavsky, 1973). Organizations, especially public agencies, are social structures characterized by fixed jurisdictions, hierarchy, and specialized expertise all designed to interpret and apply policy, and often to deliver services to clientele. The work of public organizations in giving practical meaning to statutes, or formalized policy, is neither simple nor straightforward, however. Differences in implementation strategies depend on a number of factors including tractability of the problem, design of the policy, and variables specific to the agency and the personnel assigned responsibility for program implementation.

Tractability refers to the fact that some problems are more easily remedied than others (Mazmanian & Sabatier, 1983). Factors that affect tractability include technology and problem structure itself, as well as characteristics of the population affected (Schon & Rein, 1995). Often from the perspective of those responsible for policy implementation, an optimal strategy when facing difficult problems is one of avoidance, that is, either not allowing oneself to be assigned program responsibilities or, alternatively, redesigning and redefining program objectives to reflect measurable and achievable results.

In the health field, prevention may be an optimal strategy for improving outcomes in most instances. In policy terms, however, prevention poses the greatest problem of tractability. For example, childhood immunization, an optimal strategy for dealing with many diseases, encounters intractable issues of delivery in very specific populations. As a consequence of tractability, policies dealing with health care often employ a decomposed, single-focus format narrowly formulated to address specific diseases or specific delivery problems. Broader approaches to health issues, such as prevention and promotion, encounter too many problems of tractability to build a sufficient record of success needed to secure a stable resource base and ongoing program viability.

Design variables also shape the transformation of policies into programs and services. Policy design reflects the premise that the effects of policy depend in part on how policy is organized. Well-crafted policy incorporates consideration of agency needs and guidelines, legal mandates, organizational routines, practitioner and client needs, and environmental factors (Schon & Rein, 1995). Factors most often considered as key to good design include clear and concise objectives, adequate understanding of causal effects, sufficient start-up funds and resources, coordination between responsible agencies, formalization of rules, and clear channels of communication (Schneider & Ingram, 1990). Examples of policies that fail to incorporate such considerations at the stage of design are legion.

In its present stage of development, the literature on implementation has several practical suggestions for those responsible for translating policy into programs. The most useful include the interrelated ideas of backward mapping and incorporation of the needs of "street-level bureaucrats," that is, practitioners. Backward mapping requires that the logic of policy be reversible and based on key juncture points, as well as on the practitioner's environment (Elmore, 1985). Relying on the analogy of mapping out an automobile trip from one point to another, Elmore described the logic of policy implementation: "To get from a starting point . . . to a result, . . . we don't just set an objective and go there. We begin at either end and reason both ways, back and forth, until we discover a satisfactory connection" (p. 35). Implementation cannot succeed without consideration of both starting and ending points as well as all necessary intermediate connections. Backward mapping expands the focus in implementation from the problem to be solved, to the practitioner and the environment in which services are delivered to people. Lipsky (1980) was one of the first to describe the interactive dynamics of practice on program, personnel, and policy in his research on the applied professions. He viewed policy not as the formal statements of statutes and officials but as the patterns of behavior produced by street-level bureaucrats. Again, the limits of the environment in which practitioners deliver services further condition and constrain the development of programs and must be considered as factors in designing implementation strategies.

Issues surrounding policy implementation have received little consideration in the nursing literature. Input from staff administrators on policy design and implementation has been overlooked. For example, discharge planning becomes a series of front-end loaded, prescriptive, standardized planning procedures rather than an outcomes driven, interactive process. Including an implementation perspective in discharge planning would require consideration of the problems encountered at the delivery level by both nurses and their patients. Similarly, continuity of care has become a prescriptive mantra rather than a well-understood process. Progress in this policy area cannot be made until continuity of care is viewed as a problem of implementation involving multiple organizational providers and funding sources and employing a patient/outcomes perspective.

Some progress toward consideration of issues of implementation into nursing practice is evident, although it has not yet been incorporated by nurses through a policy lens. A growing emphasis on outcomes-based strategies of care reflects a "backward mapping" approach. The broadening of thinking about nursing care strategies from front-end issues such as nursing diagnoses to back-end delivery issues, such as nursing interventions and patient outcomes, reflects a gradual incorporation of the practice environment into organizational programming.

Evaluation

The last stage in the formal model of policy making is that of evaluation. Program evaluation seeks objective information about how policies perform or whether an activity is worth doing. Evaluation is mandated with increasing frequency both as a means to monitor programs and to assess their impacts and efficiency. Evaluation generally involves several steps:

- Identification of the goals to be evaluated
- Analysis of the problems with which the activity must cope
- Standardized descriptions of program activities
- Determination of whether observed changes are attributable to the program or to another cause
- Estimation of the effects and costs (Jones, 1984, p. 210)

Program evaluation, however, is a far more complex, self-contradictory, and difficult process than current practice acknowledges. Although an important source of feedback necessary for adjusting and improving policy, evaluation actually relies far more on the political and environmental dynamics of the policy sector in which it is set than it does on a formalized, objective, and independent evaluation process. This is largely because policies and programs are delivered by organizations.

Evaluation and organization may be contradictory terms; organizational structure implies stability, but evaluation suggests change. . . . Evaluation speaks of the relationship between action and objectives, whereas organization relates its activities to programs and clientele. (Wildavsky, 1979, p. 220)

The dynamics and requirements of policy and of organizations responsible for administering policy differ. Organizations are formed to stabilize their environment, therefore enhancing predictability, fairness, and reproducibility in social interaction. Evaluation challenges basic organizational requisites and is dysfunctional from an organizational perspective. Generally, evaluation is viable only as it sustains rather than challenges organizational functions. Within these basic parameters, however, evaluation can provide useful information about the margins rather than the substantive core of policy or programmatic activities. The limits of evaluation, however, must be clearly understood (deLeon, 1988-1989).

Evaluation is first and foremost a political activity. Its purpose is to discern that knowledge about policy that enables the connection between the interests of organizational and political leaders and constituencies to be maintained. The incentive for pursuing evaluation is first to justify the legitimacy of a program's budgetary asking and, second, to allow information slowly to shape and rework formal and informal policy. However, knowledge derived from evaluation does not always result in greater agreement. Obtaining good objective information is one of the greatest challenges for public agencies. The drive for self-preservation conditions organizations to shape information derived from evaluation at all levels. This occurs through the selective management of evaluation results as they move upward through organizational hierarchies from the program to the decision-making levels (Wilensky, 1967). Again, evaluation serves both internal and external organizational agendas first and any substantive policy logic only secondarily.

Finally, timing in evaluation is key, although it is little discussed in the literature. Evaluation is frequently mandated by funding or budgetary cycles. The impact of policy initiatives, however, is rarely related to such cycles. Policy effects are often neither obvious nor direct within short time frameworks. There can be a long lag time between a policy change and any measurable impact. In addition, change can be indirect, arising from delayed, or sleeper, effects and from unanticipated consequences. Such effects often are more meaningful and far reaching but regularly missed by traditional evaluation strategies (Salamon, 1976). To illustrate, results from evaluations of nursing interventions on behalf of those acutely ill will always be more definitive and clear than those assessing prevention or health promotion. Evaluation strategies for policies affecting the latter are far more difficult to design, fund, and demonstrate. As a result, they are less likely to be performed.

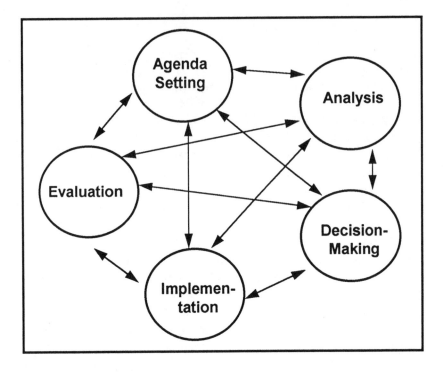

Figure 4.3: Policy Process

Summary

The policy process is usually divided into five stages and presented as a linear cycle. There is, in reality, no necessary direction or sequence in the policy process. As suggested in Figure 4.3, the process by which problems command the attention of policymakers with decisions made, implemented, and evaluated is much more interactive than linear.

Again, policy, whether incremental or comprehensive, depends on input and feedback from the environment in which it unfolds. Successful policy entrepreneurs are those persons skilled in understanding how to merge environment, process, and substance, a task dependent on multiple factors plus some luck.

HEALTH POLICY AND NURSING

Nursing policy can be viewed independently or as an emerging subset nested within the larger health policy sector. The policy literature informs both perspectives. In developing the former, however, nursing needs some understanding of the latter. The health policy sector is an increasingly crowded, interdependent, and interactive environment with its own internal dynamics. Viewing nursing both as a subset of health policy as well as its own policy sector is useful for nurses interested in policy strategy and processes. Thinking incrementally and strategically rather than globally and ideologically may in the long run be more productive for nurse activists interested in consolidating their role in the health sector.

From a policy perspective, the health sector both suffers from and capitalizes on several pathologies. Most salient among these for nursing policy is ongoing goal displacement driven, in part, by increasing problems of policy tractability. Policy objectives that prove difficult or impossible to attain in practice are replaced or revised to incorporate new goals. Health policy benefited from its early successes in limited areas of medicine and public health. Over time, as more readily treatable diseases were identified, life expectancy increased, but more complex and endemic health problems were exposed. Propelled by its successes, medical care with its episodic focus has both broadened into health care with its holistic focus and been institutionalized as policy and a public responsibility. Health, however, is a far more nebulous, subjective, and unobtainable policy goal than medical care. Next, arising from the government's assumption of responsibility for the care of the elderly and poor, health care has been institutionalized. This has added criteria of access and fairness to the policy mix. Access and fairness are criteria by which organizations, politicians, and the public measure policy outcomes. Both changes reflect goal displacement as expectations for policy evolve over time.

As goals broaden and change, however, health policy becomes less tractable. When outcomes for one set of objectives, such as access and fairness, prove difficult, if not impossible, to define and translate, the incentives for further rounds of goal displacement reappear. Cost containment, quality standards, and even decentralization of responsibility for care (Wakefield, 1995) now compete for priority as more recent entrants in the mix of health policy goals. Each round of displacement enlarges and diffuses the number and focus of policies in the health policy sector, as well as compounds problems of tractability at the stage of implementation. Goal displacement is driven partly by new players seeking to enhance their resources and roles in a policy sector. Expansion both in the number and in the level of activity of players competing for resources in the health policy sector decreases the likelihood of coherent policy change, however.

As the front-end goals of policy are displaced and become competitive with each other, then "back-end" considerations, that is the dynamics of implementation involving questions of resources and service delivery, emerge to drive the process and to allocate care. Money and the limitations of patient care delivery systems (availability, time, distance, complexity, communication, space, etc.) now ration care and provide the basic constraints that condition policy considerations in health at this time. Implementation dynamics have come to dominate a policy sector in which crowding and competing interests on one side and the infinite elasticity of demand on the other have combined to limit possibilities for coordination and agreement. Yet early arriving actors in the health policy field have preserved their base of services and resources, benefited incrementally, and can expect to maintain their position.

Nursing policy can be viewed as both a subset within the health policy sector and a separate policy arena. From the perspective of the former, nurses have firsthand knowledge derived from practice that has particular utility in informing health policy in its present phase of development. Issues of implementation now dominate the health sector. This focus on the delivery of care reflects belated attempts to reconcile the constraints and dynamics of practice settings with policy objectives. The benefits to nursing of "backward mapping"—that is, of building policy initiatives from its base of practice—provide an opportunity to secure a substantial role in the health policy arena. Effectiveness for nurses as policy entrepreneurs, however, depends on an understanding of policy processes and on disciplined strategies for achieving carefully defined, narrow, nursing objectives directed primarily on the phase of implementation, rather than on generating comprehensive reform efforts that can only contribute to further rounds of goal displacement. Being a player with the power to churn goals may appear to generate momentum at one level but often results in little meaningful change for nursing practitioners delivering care.

Nursing policy as a subset of the health policy sector may be better served with greater long-term impact by operating incrementally but systematically. That is, nurses, as first-line practitioners, are best able to identify solutions that work. The necessary next step is to attach those solutions to tractable policy problems within practice settings and then to act as policy entrepreneurs. There is some evidence that the nursing community has begun to understand this:

> The focus . . . is on the ability of the leader to create solutions. The truth is that it is easy to identify problems. The biggest and most visible agenda is to create solutions that will propel the organization forward. (Vestral, 1995, p. 86)

The policy literature is rich with descriptions of lessons learned about the dynamics of policy. This chapter has reviewed the literature on policy process for nurses interested in securing and enhancing the role of nursing in the changing health care delivery system. Nursing must incorporate this knowledge into policy initiatives. The organizational level where policy is translated into practice contains a major source of policy information for nursing. The lessons of practice are available as solutions to be attached to policy problems. Good policy design is primarily incremental in form and employs "backward-mapping" techniques. Policy is not always large in scale or scope (Beyers, 1995). Improved policy development requires systematic input from nursing administrators operating at the service delivery level. This linkage is key to better policy development. With more realistic understanding of the processes and dynamics of policy, the nursing role in the multiple levels of policy in the health care sector can become substantive rather than symbolic.

REFERENCES

Allison, G. (1971). *Essence of decision: Explaining the Cuban missile crisis.* Boston: Little, Brown.

Anderson, J. (1975). *Public policy making.* New York: Praeger.

Baumgartner, F., & Jones, B. (1993). *Agendas and instability in American politics.* Chicago: University of Chicago Press.

Beyers, M. (1995). Public policy and the nurse administrator. *Nursing Policy Forum, 1*(1), 28-33.

Braybrooke, D., & Lindblom, C. (1963). *A strategy of decision.* Glenco, NY: The Free Press.

Cohen, M., March, J., & Olsen, J. (1972). A garbage can model of organizational choice. *Administrative Science Quarterly, 17,* 1-25.

deLeon, P. (1988-1989). The contextual burdens of policy design. *Policy Studies Journal, 17*(2), 297-309.

Elmore, R. (1985). Forward and backward mapping: Reversible logic in the analysis of public policy. In K. Hanfe & T. Toonen (Eds.), *Public policy implementation in federal and unitary systems* (pp. 23-70). Dordrecht, The Netherlands: Martinus Nighoff.

Hanley, B. (1993). Policy development and analysis. In D. Mason, S. Talbott, & J. Leavitt (Eds.). *Policy and politics for nurses* (2nd ed.). Philadelphia: W. B. Saunders.

Harrington, C., & Estes, C. (Eds.). (1994). *Health policy and nursing: Crisis and reform in the U.S. health care delivery system.* Boston: Jones & Bartlett.

Heclo, H. (1975). Frontiers of social policy in Europe and America. *Policy Sciences, 6*(4), 404-413.

Helms, L. (1981). Policy analysis in education: The case for incrementalism. *Executive Review, 1*(6), 1-6. Iowa City: Institute of School Executives.

Jones, C. (1984). *An introduction to the study of public policies.* Boston: Little, Brown.

Kalisch, B., & Kalisch, P. (1982). *Politics of nursing.* Philadelphia: J. B. Lippincott.

Kingdon, J. (1984). *Agendas, alternatives & public policies.* Boston: Little, Brown.

Lescavage, R. (1995). Nurses, make your presence felt. *Nursing Policy Forum, 1*(1), 18-21.

Lindblom, C. (1979, November-December). Still muddling: Not yet through. *Public Administration Review, 39,* 517-526.

Lipsky, M. (1980). *Street level bureaucracy.* Boston: Little, Brown.

MacRae, D., & Wilde, J. (1985). *Policy analysis for public decisions.* Lanham, MD: University Press of America.

Madison, J. (1787-1788). The Federalist Papers, Numbers 10 and 51. In C. Rossiter (Ed.), *The Federalist Papers* (pp. 77-83, 320-324). New York: Mentor Books, 1961.

Mason, D., & Talbott, S. (Eds.). (1985). *Political action: Handbook for nurses.* Menlo Park, CA: Addison-Wesley.

Mason, D., Talbott, S., & Leavitt, J. (Eds.). (1993). *Policy and politics for nurses.* Philadelphia: W. B. Saunders.

Mazmanian, D., & Sabatier, P. (1983). *Implementation and public policy*. Glenview, IL: Scott Foresman.

Mitchell, P., Krueger, J., & Moody, L. (1990). The crisis of the health care nonsystem. *Nursing Outlook, 38*(5), 214-217.

O'Neill, M., & Pederson, A. (1992). Building a methods bridge between public policy analysis and health public policy. *Canadian Journal of Public Health, 83*, 825-830.

Pressman, J., & Wildavsky, A. (1973). *Implementation*. Berkeley: University of California Press.

Rains, J., & Hahn (1995). Policy research: Lessons from the field. *Public Health Nursing, 12*(2), 72-77.

Salamon, L. (1976). Follow-ups, letdowns, and sleepers: The time dimension in policy evaluation. In C. Jones & R. Thomas (Eds.), *Public policy making in a federal system* (pp. 257-384). Beverly Hills, CA: Sage.

Schneider, A., & Ingram, H. (1990). Policy design: Elements, premises and strategies. In S. Nagel (Ed.), *Policy theory and policy evaluation* (pp. 77-101). New York: Greenwood Press.

Schon, D. & Rein, M. (1995). *Frame reflection: Toward the resolution of intractable policy controversies*. New York: Basic Books.

Sochalski, J. (1993). The dynamics of public policy: A walk through the process. In D. Mason, S. Talbott, & J. Leavitt (Eds.), *Policy and politics for nurses* (2nd ed., pp. 88-103). Philadelphia: W. B. Saunders.

Stimpson, M. & Hanley, B. (1991). Nurse policy analyst: Advance practice role. *Nursing and Health Care, 12*, 10-15.

Stokey, E. & Zeckhauser, R. (1978). *A primer for policy analysis*. New York: W. W. Norton.

Vestral, K. (1995). Nurse executives: Career derailment, success, and dilemmas. *Nursing Administration Quarterly, 19*(4), 83-89.

Wakefield, M. (1995). Medicaid bloc grants: A new beginning or the end of an era. *Nursing Policy Forum, 1*(3), 4-7.

Weick, K. (1969). *The social psychology of organizing*. Reading, MA: Addison-Wesley.

Weiss, C. (1980). *Social science research and decisionmaking*. New York: Columbia University Press.

Wildavsky, A. (1979). *Speaking truth to power*. Boston: Little, Brown.

Wilensky, H. (1967). *Organizational intelligence*. New York: Basic Books.

CHAPTER 5

The Evolving Role
of the Informatics Nurse

Connie Delaney
Peg Mehmert
Dickey Johnson

The knowledge/information explosion brought about by the confluence of computers and communication technology is transforming many aspects of today's world. One manifestation of this transformation is the movement to restructure the U.S. health care system, which is being aided by an unprecedented access to health care information. Accessible information is the crucial component necessary for rational decision making about cost, quality, and access to health services for individuals, groups, and organizations. The informatics nurse, who is uniquely trained to integrate computer science, information science, and nursing science, has the special knowledge, technical skills, and vision to produce computerized information systems that reflect and support nursing practice, thereby enabling the nurse executive and the nursing profession to achieve goals such as improved service, higher quality of care, and increased cost effectiveness. Over the last three decades, nursing informatics has gradually grown into a complex and multifaceted specialty in which informatics nurses participate proactively in standardized language development, in needs assessment, and in systems planning, design, development, implementation, and evaluation. Their role cuts across all three principal aspects of health care reform, including restructuring, redesign, and reengineering. This chapter examines the evolving role of the informatics nurse and considers some implications for nurse administrators regarding effective management of that role.

The Information Age is here. The phenomenal confluence of computers and communication technology that has occurred in the 20th century has made it possible for information to be readily stored, processed, and shared, making it accessible in ways previously impossible. As our society creates wealth and power based on the use of knowledge as the raw material, the resulting knowledge and information explosion is transforming groups, organizations, networks, systems, and the world.

One manifestation of this transformation is the movement to restructure the U.S. system of health care. The call for reform permeates health care agendas in both public and private services, sites, and settings. Although multiple energies contribute to health care reform, accessibility to health information is the linchpin that makes the reform movement possible. Accessible information is the crucial component necessary for rational decision making about cost, quality, and access to health services for individuals, groups, and organizations.

Members of the nursing profession, who have always stood as key advocates for consumers of health care, have a vital role to play in ensuring that information-driven health care delivery systems ultimately benefit the consumer. Informatics nurses, in particular, focus on making computerized health care facts (i.e., data) available, valid, and simple and work to ensure that interpretation of those facts (i.e., information) will result in improved coordination of care, higher quality of care, and increased cost effectiveness. It is incumbent on nurse administrators, meanwhile, to understand the vital role of the informatics nurse so that the administrators will find the resources to support the informatics role, position the informatics nurse effectively within the organization, and empower informatics nurses to represent nursing on the interdisciplinary information management teams.

An informatics nurse is a nurse specialist who holds a master's degree in nursing, which includes advanced education in nursing, leadership development, and research, and has taken graduate-level courses in the fields of information management and computer science. Uniquely trained to integrate these three areas—computer science, information science, and nursing science—the informatics nurse has the special knowledge and leadership skills to assess the information needs not only of clinical nurses but also of nurse administrators, nurse educators, and nurse researchers and the vision to design, implement, and maintain an information system that reflects and supports nursing practice, rather than a system that forces nurses to conform to technology. By designing an information system that focuses on client care, for example, the informatics nurse helps clinical nurses and nurse administrators deliver client care more effectively. Meanwhile, the same system, if well designed, can simultaneously support nursing research (e.g., by providing for the development of a clinical database, with checks to ensure the validity and reliability of the data) and nursing education (e.g., by incorporating decision-making algorithms that facilitate clinical decision making at levels ranging from student novice to expert).

Because of their unique training and skills, informatics nurses can and do serve in various positions throughout the nursing profession. They can be consultants, system analysts, information coordinators, nursing information specialists, resource managers, directors of informatics, or designers of information systems and software. Regardless of the position or the setting— whether in homes, commercial businesses, information systems departments, or at the bedside in institutions—the fundamental role of the informatics nurse is to provide clinicians, providers, and consumers with the data and information they need to make health care decisions that are consistent with the goals of improved service, quality of care, and cost effectiveness.

To perform this role well, informatics nurses cannot simply acknowledge information technology, as nurses generally did in the past. Informatics nurses today must proactively foster participation in the development and use of a standardized language about nursing diagnoses, interventions, and outcomes. They must become adept at strategic planning and assessment of user needs. They must become experts in the design and development of computerized information systems—in selecting, testing, implementing, maintaining, and evaluating systems and in training others to use the systems. Moreover, they must be cognizant of the social, political, ethical, and legal environments in which they are working because these can influence every aspect of information management, such as the effective implementation and ongoing use of the systems they design.

Thus, the scope of practice of the informatics nurse today encompasses a skilled and dynamic approach to the use of information systems. This chapter examines the evolving role of the informatics nurse and considers some implications for nurse administrators regarding effective management of that role. The first section defines and discusses the historical development of nursing informatics as a specialty within nursing. The next section describes the characteristics and competencies of the informatics nurse. The last section analyzes the ongoing role of the informatics nurse as it cuts across all three principal aspects of health care reform: restructuring (system or organizational architecture), redesign (who should be doing what), and reengineering (the process of how things are accomplished).

EVOLUTION OF THE ROLE

Nursing's Entry into Computerized Information Technology

The application of computerized information technology to health care began in the 1960s and 1970s. Most early information systems were primarily in-house projects, usually focused on either management, financial, admission, discharge, and transfer (ADT) information, or order entry and results reporting. Nurses rarely assisted with the design of these initial health care computing applications. If nursing was involved in these early efforts, it was primarily in the provision of staff education and training.

As information systems moved to include clinical data, however, nurses—who are at the hub of collecting, sharing, and using clinical data—became more active. Margo Cook, RN, and Donna McNeill, RN, in the El Camino Hospital project in Mountain View, California, were among the first nurses to assist in the design and development of a hospital information system with clinical applications (Cook & McDowell, 1975). They participated not only in defining the content and designing the function of an information system for a nursing unit but also in implementing and evaluating the system. Another early example of nursing input can be found at the Latter Day Saints (LDS) Hospital in Salt Lake City, Utah. There a clinical user group participated in the design and development of ICU functions, computer-generated protocols, and evaluation of computer applications to alert clinicians to abnormal laboratory values. Other early nursing efforts to develop clinical systems occurred at the Charlotte Memorial Hospital in Charlotte, North Carolina (Sommers, 1971), and at the Medical Center of Vermont, where the innovative Problem Oriented Medical Information System (which has subsequently served as one of the Institute of Medicine's models for computer-based patient records) was developed (Weed, 1969).

Nurses' satisfaction with these early systems was marginal. This limited satisfaction can be attributed to several factors. First, the early systems were usually adapted from systems focused on financial functions, which meant that although they were generally proficient in handling quantitative data, they were often inefficient and ineffective in accommodating clinical patient care data, which can be more qualitative, voluminous, and subject to finer shades of meaning. Second, early implementation efforts typically failed to involve clinicians/users in the design and development phases, so input from users was indirect or intermittent. The resulting applications tended, therefore, to be inadequate to meet the varied and complex needs of different patient populations or diverse information requirements of various areas within the health care institutions. Third, the software engineers and computer programmers (systems analysts) associated with the early information systems rarely had the knowledge base necessary to identify the complex needs of the health care system, its managers, and a variety of clinicians. Their lack of knowledge limited the functionality of the systems they designed, especially with regard to user interfaces and reports. Fourth, nurses involved in system development were working in isolation from one another, with no professional organized structure to facilitate networking. The lack of publications and educational opportunities hampered nurses' ability to learn more sophisticated system analysis, design, and implementation techniques from experts in the field and apply that knowledge to meet their needs.

Three factors—the increasing complexity inherent in nursing practice, the volume of information managed by nurses, and the need to meet government and nongovernment mandated standards in health care—were driving forces in a variety of initiatives that eventually led to the identification of clinical data elements, the development of nursing information systems, and the recognition of nursing informatics as a specialty in nursing. Responding to the need to computerize nursing data at St. Louis University, Gebbie and Lavin (1975) convened the First National Conference for the Classification of Nursing Diagnoses in 1974. The focus of this first conference was to identify patient conditions that were amenable to nursing intervention. The conference thus represented the first attempt to develop a standardized language to describe the problems that nurses treat in a manner that allows the information to be easily encoded in computers. The development of standardized language continued from this early work and now encompasses not only nursing diagnoses but also nursing interventions, outcomes, and management variables (McCormick et al., 1994).

Major Initiatives within the Nursing Profession

By the late 1970s, the necessity for developing nursing information systems had gained national attention. A national conference on nursing information systems, organized in 1977 by Werley and Grier (1981), explored "the state of the art in defining and using nursing information systems that articulate with medical and health agency information systems" (p. ix). Further, through a national conference in 1985, nursing experts reached consensus regarding the elements composing a Nursing Minimum Data Set (NMDS) (Werley & Lang, 1988).

Professional nursing associations have supported the progress in developing, implementing, and evaluating nursing information systems, fostering networking, and providing educational opportunities and resources for informatics nurses. The American Nurses Association (ANA), for example, established the Council on Computer Applications in 1984 and endorsed the NMDS in 1986 (Zielstorff, Hudgings, & Grobe, 1993; Zielstorff, McHugh, & Clinton, 1988). Realizing the imperative for standardizing nursing language, ANA created the ANA Steering Committee on Databases to Support Clinical Nursing Practice in 1989. This committee addresses professional policy and initiatives for developing nursing classifications, uniform data sets, and national databases; building clinical data sets; and coordinating public and private initiatives in database development. Four classification systems have already been recommended by the ANA Steering Committee for inclusion in national databases: (a) the North American Nursing Diagnosis Association (NANDA) Taxonomy of Nursing Diagnoses, (b) the Nursing Interventions Classification (NIC), (c) the Omaha Community Health Problem and Intervention Classification System, and (d) the Home Health Care Classification. Extensive development has subsequently occurred on another classification system, the Nursing-Sensitive Outcomes Classification (NOC), and on another minimum data set, the Nursing Management Minimum Data Set (NMMDS), although these have not yet been recommended by the ANA Steering Committee (Gardner, Delaney, Crossley, Mehmert, & Ellerbe, 1992; McCormick et al., 1994).

Further, ANA collaborated with the National League for Nursing Informatics Forum and the National Commission on Nursing Implementation Project to promote dialogue that resulted in identifying criteria for state-of-the-art information systems. Essentials for these systems are summarized in the *Computer Design Criteria* (Zielstorff, McHugh, & Clinton, 1988) and the *Next-Generation Nursing Information Systems* (Zielstorff, Hudgings, & Grobe, 1993). These publications include guidelines for nurses and vendors regarding the development of information systems to support nursing practice within the context of a total, integrated, computer-based patient record. Most recently, ANA (1994) published the *Scope of Practice for Nursing Informatics* and implemented a certification exam for this specialty area. The ANA is also collaborating with the International Council of Nurses' initiative to develop an international classification for nursing practice, which expands efforts to define nursing data and standardize its language to the international level (International Council of Nurses, 1993).

Other professional organizational support for nursing informatics has come from the American Organization of Nurse Executives (AONE) and the National League for Nursing. For example, AONE, which is committed to identifying and meeting the data needs of nurse managers and executives, supports the work of Gardner-Huber, Delaney, and associates to define and test a nursing management minimum data set ("Advisory board appointed," 1996; "AONE joins with the University of Iowa," 1996; Gardner et al., 1992). The National League for Nursing, meanwhile, has recognized the imperative of preparing graduates with a background in computers and information systems (Peterson & Gerdin-Jelger, 1988).

The proliferation of publications and professional education programs related to nursing informatics has fostered collegial exchange and the growth of expertise in nursing information systems. Building on the newsletter format first published in 1983, the first journal specifically focusing on computers in nursing, *Computers in Nursing*, was published in 1984 (Saba & McCormick, 1986). Sigma Theta Tau International has continued to place high priority on advancing nursing's knowledge base by using the advantages of the electronic medium. Clear evidence of this is the creation of nursing's first electronic journal, *The Online Journal of Knowledge Synthesis for Nursing* (Barnsteiner, 1994). Professional nursing education programs in nursing informatics were implemented at the baccalaureate, master's, and doctoral levels in the late 1980s and early 1990s. Continuing education programs focusing on all aspects of computers and the use of information systems in all practice settings have been established. Finally, the development of the informatics agenda by the National Institute for Nursing Research (National Center for Nursing Research, 1993) further illustrates nursing's responsiveness to the data-driven paradigm shift that is propelling us into the 21st century.

Nursing's Response to External Mandates

External mandates have also increased the urgency of nursing's response and participation in the development of computerized information systems. For example, the Joint Commission on the Accreditation of Health Care Organizations (JCAHO, 1994) formally required nursing's participation in systems selection, design, and implementation and in the evaluation of the standards for information management. As a result of that mandate, hospitals have included nurse managers, nurse administrators, and informatics nurse specialists as full-fledged members of information management committees, rather than simply as occasional consultants.

In a similar vein, the Institute of Medicine (IOM) has strongly encouraged participation of nurses and inclusion of nursing data in its initiative to develop a nationwide computer-based patient record (CPR): a birth-to-death, totally electronic, health care record that is accessible across all health care delivery sites and settings and to all health care providers, consumers, and payers (IOM, 1991). Nurses serve on several critical IOM committees, including the Codes and Structure Workgroup Executive Committee, the Committee for Improving the Patient Record in Response to Increasing Functional Requirements and Technological Advances, the Users and Uses Subcommittee, and the Technology Subcommittee.

Summary: From Reactive to Proactive

Over the past three decades, nursing has moved from a position of minimal involvement and passive response to computer applications to its current proactive stance. This stance strongly supports nursing informatics endeavors that focus on the data and information needs of the profession for the provision of patient care. Nursing has become actively involved in developing language to support computerizing clinical data. Through continuing education and formal educational opportunities, a growing cadre of informatics nurses has developed expertise in identifying clinical information needs and participating in systems planning, design, development, implementation, and evaluation. Graduates at all levels of nursing education are acquiring computer skills that allow them to be informed users. Professional associations, informatics literature, informatics research priorities, and ongoing educational opportunities now support broader networking, the sharing and development of knowledge, and active participation in nursing information systems.

CHARACTERISTICS AND COMPETENCIES
OF THE INFORMATICS NURSE

As nursing's engagement with information technologies has evolved and deepened, the characteristics and competencies needed by the informatics nurse have taken on a definitive shape. It is clear that to promote the effective and efficient use of data and information by nurse managers, administrators, and staff, the informatics nurse needs knowledge of computers and technology, information management, and nursing science. Specifically, the informatics nurse needs conceptual knowledge about (a) how to analyze information needs and design computerized systems to respond to those needs (system design and analysis); (b) how to identify what pieces of information (facts) are relevant, and how those pieces relate to each other (data structures and databases); and (c) how individual workstations are linked together to facilitate the exchange of information among various sites and users (networks and distributed systems). Moreover, the informatics nurse needs the technical skill to apply that conceptual knowledge to the nursing experience, that is, for example, to make judgments about which computer hardware and software applications will be most suitable, to determine how to install a given application or decision-support system, to develop maintenance procedures and schedules, and to decide what aspects of performance must be evaluated and when.

The informatics nurse's content knowledge and technical skills are insufficient, however, unless they are also balanced with skills in leadership, education, and research processes and an appreciation of the social, political, ethical, and legal environments in which specific information systems are developed and used. Ultimately, the informatics nurse works not simply with data but also with people: as individuals, within organizations, and within the larger health care systems. The values of those individuals, organizations, and systems determine what technologies are developed, what characteristics they will have, and how they will be used. In turn, all technologies, including information systems, convey value back onto individuals, organizations, and systems. That is, all technologies are based on specific assumptions, confer benefit(s) on certain individuals or groups, and are expressions (at least in some ways) of individual preferences, tastes, worldviews, cultural values, and political goals (McGinn, 1990).

For example, the specific values of nurse managers and administrators—regarding centralized versus decentralized decision making, levels of trust, or lines of authority, for instance—influence not only what data or information are available to whom, when, and for what purposes but also the future expression of values within the work environment. A department of nursing that values shared governance might have no hesitation in sharing data regarding costs of care or staff/patient ratios with staff nurses, whereas a department of nursing that maintains centralized decision making or has low levels of trust is likely to limit staff access to such information. In the first case, access to the technology and data confers benefit onto the staff nurse and can increase responsibility, accountability, and participation in the shared governance model; limited access to the data, meanwhile, can lead to further lack of staff participation, reinforcing the need for centralized decision making. In either case, the role of the informatics nurse would be the same: to raise responsibly questions and support deliberations about what data are collected, how they are collected, for what purposes they are collected, how they are shared, with whom they are shared, and how they are used. Thus, the informatics nurse helps the patients, the practitioners, and the administrators of the health care system face the issues inherent in an information-driven society and balance their needs within the context of the strengths and limitations of the technology and the financial resources of all of those involved.

Overall, the responsibility and accountability for system design, development, and implementation places the informatics nurse in an innovative and rewarding role that supports "development and evaluation of applications, tools, processes, and structures that assist nurses with the management of data in taking care of patients or supporting the practice of nursing" (ANA, 1994, p. 3). Although the role demands certain characteristics and competencies, ultimately the effectiveness of informatics nurses hinges on the ability to view the needs of nursing from both the macro perspective of the organization and the integrated perspective of an entire health care delivery system. The role may be an isolated position filled with the constant pressures of being a change agent, yet that isolation is increasingly counterbalanced by the opportunity to interact with other staff across disciplines, departmental boundaries, practice sites, and settings and by support within the nursing profession and departments of nursing in the form of newsletters, other educational resources, networking, and conferences.

THE ROLE OF THE INFORMATICS NURSE
IN CHANGING HEALTH CARE

The availability of the informatics nurse and the evolution of information systems have already started transforming the health care delivery system by bringing about changes in the organizational structure of health care delivery institutions (restructuring), changes in who should be doing what (redesign), and changes in how things are done within those institutions (reengineering). For example, most health care organizations that have some type of computerized information system(s) in place have achieved more efficient levels of financial accounting and claims processing. These organizations have also streamlined communication among health care services, such as ordering laboratory tests and obtaining the results (IOM, 1991).

The future impact of these information technologies on the restructuring, redesign, and reengineering of health care delivery, however, is directly related to the quality and the capabilities of the technologies that are used. Simpson (1995) noted that although 99% of hospitals use financial systems, only 14% have point-of-care documentation and less than 9% have clinical data repositories. Thus, only a handful have acquired state-of-the-art systems capable of serving the changes required in an integrated health care delivery system that is being reformed. Most institutions still find themselves in the awkward position of having spent millions of dollars on information systems that satisfactorily handle their financial management needs but fail to address the need to manage and process clinical information. Numerous institutions, therefore, are in the process of evaluating their current systems and asking the questions: "What can we salvage?" "What do we need to replace?" "What do we look for?"

There is no lack of answers to these questions. A wide range of health care experts, including hospital administrators, nursing executives, informatics nurses, and clinicians have suggested the form that information systems must take to meet the requirements of health care reform: They must be integrated, community-based, multi-institutional systems that can accommodate an interdisciplinary approach to health care, streamline the delivery process, facilitate multitasking of health care roles, support data repositories, incorporate outcome-based quality care measurements, enhance cost containment, and increase data availability across all encounters (IOM, 1991). To acquire or develop these clinically oriented systems, institutions must have the financial means, of course, but they also require access to informatics nurses to help develop the system as well as nursing administrators who understand the needs of the staff, the clients, the organization, and the health care delivery system and who appreciate the informatics nurse's role in addressing those needs.

The informatics nurse, whether employed within the organization or contracted through a vendor, plays a vital role in supporting nursing administrators and ensuring that the information technologies that are being put into place can and do meet these requirements. The following sections provide examples of the potential of information systems and informatics nurses to contribute to further restructuring, redesign, and reengineering of the health care delivery system.

Restructuring

Restructuring, or changing the system or organizational architecture of a health care institution, is an internal change typically motivated by a desire to increase the profit margin or contain cost. In and of itself, restructuring rarely arises from a direct motive to benefit patients.

Nevertheless, restructuring can result in more efficient delivery of health care services to clients. For example, creating integrated information systems that cross organization boundaries, divisions, and facilities opens up the possibility of reducing organizational barriers to care delivery. Integrated systems, rather than focusing on acute care departmental operations, can accommodate health care delivery changes that are becoming more client-focused, wellness-oriented, population-committed, and life span accountable. Access to client information can create a more client-centered holistic picture, rather than offering merely a snapshot of individual providers interacting sporadically with the client. Information systems can support integrated services such as acute care, home care, and wellness-oriented data sources, such as neighborhood nutrition centers and residential retirement centers. Data and information on aggregates can be retrieved from data repositories. Health information can be available and accessible across geographical boundaries and different service settings throughout the life span of individuals, families, and communities. Consequently, employing or consulting with an informatics nurse who focuses on development of an integrated information system can help nurse executives ensure that the system reaches its maximum potential.

The linkage of information systems to create community health information networks and community health management information systems also has potential to improve health care delivery. McDonald and Blum (1992) suggested that future health computing systems can, indeed must, support navigational, referential, decision-support, and programming transparency. That is, systems must support easy user access, provide alternative information sources that allow users to determine the credibility of information, provide background logic for decision support, and allow the user to examine the programming supporting system functions.

Throughout these many efforts to restructure health care institutions, informatics nurses can facilitate the development of user-friendly, efficient applications. The majority of information systems are customized to the specific organization. The informatics nurse is integrally involved in analyzing the roles, responsibilities, and information needs of the organization and ensuring that the critical information is available to health care management to support decision making. Vendors and informatics nurses can also foresee how the functionality of a system will influence the final product design/customization.

Redesign

Redesign looks at who should be doing what. Nurse managers, administrators, and policymakers who are interested in improving health care delivery, quality of care, and cost effectiveness by reexamining who is doing what can use the expertise of informatics nurses and the capabilities of well-designed computerized information management systems to help make data-based decisions regarding the appropriate use of personnel. For example, research that analyzes the Nursing Interventions Classification (NIC) interventions and activities to determine which are appropriate for unlicensed personnel and that calculates the frequency of performance for each of these interventions and activities can assist the nurse manager in deciding whether unlicensed personnel can be used on a particular unit (Iowa Intervention Project, 1996). If the unlicensed personnel are appropriate, the determination of the numbers of unlicensed personnel needed can be accurately calculated from the frequency of interventions and activities documented.

Redesign also includes the issue of determining when the data analysis needs of the organization should be subcontracted to external vendors or completed internally. A great deal has been learned about the relative merits of where the informatics nurse is placed within the organizational structure and the role the nurse administrator plays in determining effective placement. In general, the two options available to informatics nurses include (a) being employed within the health care institution or (b) contracting from without through the services of a vendor of information technologies. A nursing administrator who is conversant with the strengths and limitations inherent in these two options is in a better position to advocate the placement most appropriate for the administrator's institution and to facilitate the work of the informatics nurse.

Internal Assignment

Most health care organizations have both nursing services and information systems departments. Although the role of the informatics nurse is integral to both departments, the informatics nurse typically reports to one or the other of these departments. Positions within the nursing department can include director of information systems, project coordinator, nursing educator, manager of nursing information systems, director of nursing administration/ financial systems, or clinical information nurse specialist. Positions reporting within the information systems department can include clinical analyst, director of hospital information systems, project manager, or programmer.

Assignment of the informatics nurse to the nursing department, or to the information systems department, carries advantages and disadvantages in either case. Assignment to the department of nursing can offer greater credibility with nurses but can diminish the nurse's opportunity to have a broad overview of the organizational mission and required information system functions. Assignment within the information system department, meanwhile, can facilitate accessibility to system resources to make changes, but it can be perceived as a loss of commitment to nursing or a lack of credibility from a clinical perspective, and it can generate role conflict. The assignment must be carefully determined so that the structure most supportive of the work and responsibilities of the informatics nurse is selected. Whether placed within nursing or within information systems, the informatics nurse must be empowered and supported by both the organization's nursing administration and information technology staff.

External Assignment

Some informatics nurses are employed not by the health care institution but by computing vendors that work with the institution. Although they can work closely with the institution, and though most of their responsibilities and functions are comparable to those of informatics nurses employed within the organization, these external informatics nurses are ultimately accountable to their primary employer, the vendor, not to the institution. This situation brings advantages and disadvantages of its own. Because they are employed by a vendor interested in defining the needs of the user as precisely as possible to sell their products and service, the vendor-supplied informatics nurse is likely to be keenly committed to determining and meeting the needs of the organization.

Vendor-based informatics nurses can also handle several additional responsibilities with the vendor, which in turn can affect the strengths and limitations they bring to the institution. For example, in small companies, an informatics nurse may perform many functions, from product development and quality assurance to sales, marketing, training, and product support, whereas in larger companies, the nurse's expertise may be limited to one product or one function. Thus, the institution's nurse administrator must realize that external informatics nurses can vary in their ability to evaluate the suitability and performance of particular products, to discuss overall options, and to facilitate product integration for the health care organization.

Furthermore, hiring an external informatics nurse may not eliminate the decision regarding placement of that individual within the health care organization. Will the primary point of contact for the vendor-supplied informatics nurse be the health care institution's information systems department or its nursing services department? As discussed earlier, the nurse administrator's decision regarding this question can influence how the information system is designed, implemented, maintained, and evaluated.

Reengineering

In contrast with restructuring and redesign, the central focus of reengineering is to improve patient care delivery. Reengineering is customer driven and encompasses an analysis of the process of how things are accomplished. Reengineering is the "power of modern information systems to radically redesign our business processes to achieve dramatic improvements in their performance" (Hammer, 1990, p. 104). Simpson claims that at the crux of reengineering is the "belief that technology can help alleviate many inefficiencies and redundancies that erode patient care and profitability alike" (Simpson, 1995, p. 31). Reengineering requires looking outside and beyond the 1990s, beyond the way things have always been done, to consider how information technologies can make substantial improvements in the way information is handled. Concurrently cost and quality improvement must be priorities. Information technologies of the next century will include easier ways to access information and new communications technologies that will change the way people interact, form teams, and share information.

General Organizational Examples

Installation of a computerized information system into a health care organization will, by its very nature, reengineer the process of care delivery, whether planned or serendipitous. Computerizing a care plan, for example, and making it instantly available to the entire gamut of the health care team can streamline the communication of that plan among the members, even altering how and when the plan is used and by whom.

Creating and accessing multidisciplinary databases can further revolutionize health care delivery. When all members of the health care team, both internal and external to the organization, can share the same clinical information, such as health history, physical assessment, plan of care, and claims data, the care that is delivered can be better coordinated. This care can also be delivered at lower cost by eliminating redundant data. Shared access can facilitate care delivery across different settings, such as acute care, home care, outpatient care, rehabilitation facilities, and wellness centers. It can minimize the overhead for claims processing and enhance the availability of comparative data by provider, institution, region, and other dimensions.

Other examples of reengineering include more efficient use of the information system, including direct medication order entry by physicians (Tonges & Lawrenz, 1993). Studies of direct medication order entry systems have shown reduced risk of error, accelerated communication, increased physician and nurse convenience, and time savings. Electronic access to literature databases from the point of care helps the practitioner provide the most up-to-date research-based practice.

Finally, current experiments in virtual medicine contribute to a reengineering of how health care is being delivered (Galvin, D'Alessandro, Erkonen, Lacey, & Santer, 1994; Kienzle et al., 1995). The use of "virtual" groups or project, clinical, or research teams, for instance, promotes team work by using communications technology to provide the opportunity for nonphysical meetings. Reengineering that includes state-of-the-art communication systems opens up the possibility of pre- and postoperative teaching in the home without the need for either the patient or the practitioner to travel, the arrangement of staff meetings without the need for congruent schedules, and the opportunity for patients' families to provide direct support to the patient regardless of geographical distance.

Nursing Examples

Computerized information technology offers the capability of access to vast amounts of detailed clinical nursing data. Applying analytical methods to this vast repository of clinical data has the potential to influence the process of nursing care. Access to the Nursing Minimum Data Set (NMDS), which incorporates NANDA, NIC, and NOC, and to the Nursing Management Minimum Data Set (NMMDS) provides an unprecedented opportunity to reengineer nursing practice (Ryan & Delaney, 1995, Iowa Outcomes Project, in press):

> We (nursing) can describe "What Works?" because we have NIC and NOC. The What is NIC. The Works of What Works is NOC. With NANDA, NIC, and NOC, we can describe What Works for Whom? NANDA is the Whom. But to study What Works for Whom under what Conditions, we need the NMMDS. (J. McCLoskey, personal communication, June 19, 1996)

If informatics nurses have been involved in system design and selection and have incorporated the NMDS and the NMMDS into the system, they can ensure the capturing and archiving of essential nursing data. Professional nursing practice decisions can then be driven by data compilation, comparison, analysis, selection of interventions, and evaluation of the effects on client care.

NMDS research is demonstrating the strength of the NMDS to support data-based decision making (Delaney, 1996b; Delaney & Mehmert, 1990, 1991; Delaney, Mehmert, Prophet, & Crossley, 1994; Delaney & Moorhead, 1995; Ryan & Delaney, 1995). Nursing practice can be described using the NMDS. For example, analysis of 4,248 patient discharge records from a 250-bed community hospital over a six-month period demonstrated that nurses identified 16,142 diagnoses with 29,680 associated nursing outcomes and 191,256 interventions. The nine most frequently occurring nursing diagnoses accounted for 85% of all nursing diagnoses. Demographic profiles have been created for approximately one fourth of the NANDA diagnoses. Nursing care profiles for most frequently occurring Diagnostic Related Groups (DRGs) and medical diagnostic categories have been identified. Nursing care costs have been determined for the most frequently occurring DRGs. In a capitated health care financing arena, access to information quantifying nursing's contribution to cost for specific patient populations can assist the organization in contract bidding.

SUMMARY

In just a few decades, nursing has moved from little to no involvement in computers and information systems to a declared informatics specialty in the profession. The role of the informatics nurse spans clinical practice, management and administration, and research; informatics nurses are present within the health care institutions as well as the vendor community. Although embracing advanced technology, informatics nurses are committed to improving the delivery of health care to the client. The integral and key positioning of informatics nurses can help ensure continued access to the data, information, and knowledge required to meet the challenges of providing service, increasing the quality of care, and maintaining cost effectiveness within a seamless health care delivery system.

What lies ahead? Clearly, the computerized patient record linked to libraries, clinical practice guidelines, and other information sources will redefine what it means to deliver, monitor, and improve quality care. Multimedia health records will challenge the definition of "documentation," the meaning of standardized language, and the role of client/patient, particularly as it relates to increased participation in the plan of care through shared decision making and increased knowledge regarding informed consent decisions. Professional health care providers from multiple disciplines working on interdisciplinary health care teams to provide population-based health care will challenge traditionally guarded interorganizational communication, the interrelationship of clinical data and financial data, and the relationship between clinical data and performance appraisal and compensation. The proliferation of informatics positions raises questions regarding informatics expertise: How will enough informatics experts be educated? How much expertise does any one health care professional need?

Nursing executives need to be knowledgeable about information technology and its potential; accept, if not embrace, the technology to restructure, redesign, and reengineer health care delivery; and prepare proactively and skillfully to balance the use of technology with the human aspects of health care. In the future, care delivery will be influenced by the availability of vast amounts of information to those providing health care, the emphasis on knowledge management and access to expertise to improve care, the use of complex analytical methods to direct decision making, and the speed and free flow of information across geographic boundaries (Davenport & Short, 1990). How will nursing build and transmit knowledge? How will organizational charts of the future be configured? Will new collaborative models among nursing practice, administration, research, and education be needed? Nursing managers and administrators working in collaboration with the informatics nurses can proactively redirect the exciting health care reforms made possible by powerful information systems.

Ultimately nurse executives who are self-critical will recognize and promote appropriate technology. As Druegson (1990) asserted, technology and information systems must promote a sense of community, vitality, and communication links to every area of human endeavor. Appropriate technology will preserve diversity, promote environmental and energy balance by weighing all costs, and truly promote human health.

REFERENCES

Advisory board appointed to begin planning process for Nursing Management Minimum Data Set. (1996). *AONE News Update, 2*(10), pp. 1-2.

American Nurses Association. (1994). *The scope of practice for nursing informatics.* Washington, DC: ANA.

AONE joins with the University of Iowa to develop a Nursing Management Minimum Data Set. (1996, January 26). *AONE News Update, 2*(2), p. 1.

Barnsteiner, J. (1994). The Online Journal of Knowledge Synthesis For Nursing. *Reflections, 20*(2), 10-11.

Cook, M., & McDowell, W. (1975). Changing to an automated information system. *American Journal of Nursing, 75*(1), 46-51.

Davenport, T., & Short, J. (1990, Summer). The new industrial engineering: Information technology and business process redesign. *Sloan Management Review,* 11-27.

Delaney, C. (1996a). Significance of the nursing minimum data set for decision support in acute care. In B. Heller, M. Mills, & C. Romano (Eds.), *Information management: Strategies and support for data driven decisions in nursing and health care* (pp. 21-38). West Dundee, IL: S-N Publications.

Delaney, C. (1996b). Use of nursing informatics in advanced nursing practice roles for building healthier populations. *Journal for Advanced Nursing Quarterly, 1*(4), 48-53.

Delaney, C., & Mehmert, P. (1990). Electronic transfer of clinical NMDS facilitates nursing diagnoses validation. In R. Miller (Ed.), *Proceedings of the Fourteenth Annual Symposium on Computer Applications in Medical Care (SCAMC)* (pp. 899-901). Washington, DC: IEEE Computer Society Press.

Delaney, C., & Mehmert, P. (1991). Utility of NMDS in validation of computerized nursing diagnoses. In R. Carroll-Johnson (Ed.), *Classification of nursing diagnoses: Proceedings of the Ninth Annual North American Nursing Diagnosis Association* (pp. 175-179). Philadelphia: J. B. Lippincott.

Delaney, C., Mehmert, P., Prophet, C., & Crossley, J. (1994). Establishment of the research value of nursing minimum data set. In S. Grobe (Ed.), *Proceedings of the Fifth International Conference on Nursing Use of Computers and Information Science* (pp. 169-173). San Antonio, TX: International Medical Informatics Association.

Delaney, C., & Moorhead, S. (1995). The nursing minimum data set, standardized language, & health care quality. *Journal of Nursing Care Quality, 10*(1), 16-30.

Druegson, A. (1990). Four philosophies of technology. In L. Hickman (Ed.), *Technology as a human affair* (pp. 25-39). New York: McGraw-Hill.

Galvin, J., D'Alessandro, M., Erkonen, W., Lacey, D., & Santer, D. (1994). Virtual hospital: A link between academia and practice. *Academic Medicine, 69*(2), 130.

Gardner, Delaney, Crossley, Mehmert, & Ellerbe. (1992). A nursing management minimum data set: Significance and development. *Journal of Nursing Administration, 22*(7/8), 35-40.

Gebbie, K., & Lavin, M. (1975). *Classification of nursing diagnoses: Proceedings of the First National Conference.* St. Louis: C.V. Mosby.

Hammer, M. (1990). Reengineering work: Don't automate, obliterate. *Harvard Business Review, 68*(4), 104-112.

Iowa Intervention Project (1996). McCloskey, J. C., & Bulechek, G. M. (Eds.), *Nursing Intervention Classification (NIC)* (2nd ed.). St. Louis: Mosby-Year Book.

Iowa Outcomes Project (in press). Johnson, M., & Maas, M. (Eds.), *Nursing Outcomes Classification.* St. Louis: Mosby.

Institute of Medicine. (1991). *The computer-based patient record: An essential technology for health care.* Washington, DC: National Academy Press.

International Council of Nurses. (1993). *Nursing's next advances: An international classification for nursing practices (ICNP).* Geneva, Switzerland: ICN.

Joint Commission on the Accreditation of Health Care Organizations (JCAHO). (1994). *1995 comprehensive accreditation manual for hospitals.* Oakbrook, IL: JCAHO.

Kienzle, M., Curry, D., Franken, E. Jr., Galvin, J., Hoffman, E., Holtum, E., Shope, L., Torner, J., & Wakefield, D. (1995). Iowa's national laboratory for the study of rural telemedicine: Description of work in progress. *Bulletin of the Medical Library Association, 83*(1), 37-41.

McCormick, K., Lang, N., Zielstorff, R., Milholland, K., Saba, V., & Jacox, A. (1994). Toward standard classification schemes for nursing language: Recommendations of the American Nurses Association Steering Committee on Databases to Support Clinical Practice. *Journal of the American Medical Informatics Association, 1*(6), 421-427.

McDonald, M., & Blum, H. (1992). *Health in the information age: The emergence of health oriented telecommunication applications.* Berkeley, CA: Environmental Science & Policy Institute.

McGinn, R. (1990). What is technology? In L. Hickman (Ed.), *Technology: A human affair* (pp. 10-24). New York: McGraw-Hill.

National Center for Nursing Research. (1993). *Nursing informatics: Enhancing patient care. A report of the NCNR Priority Expert Panel on Nursing Informatics.* Bethesda, MD: US DHHH.

Peterson, H., & Gerdin-Jelger, V. (1988). *Preparing nurses for information systems: Recommended informatics competencies.* New York: NLN Publication No. 14-2234.

Ryan, P., & Delaney, C. (1995). The nursing minimum data set: Research findings and future directions. In J. J. Fitzpatrick & J. S. Stevenson (Eds.), *Annual Review of Nursing Research* (Vol. 13, pp. 169-194). New York: Springer.

Saba, V., & McCormick, K. (1986). *Essentials of computers for nurses.* Philadelphia: J. B. Lippincott.

Simpson, R. (1995). Reengineering: Embracing technology to improve patient care. *Nursing Management, 1,* 31-33.

Sommers, J. (1971). A computerized nursing care system. *Hospitals, 45*(8), 93-100.

Tonges, M., & Lawrenz, E. (1993). Reengineering: The work redesign-technology link. *Journal of Nursing Administration, 23*(10), 15-22.

Weed, L. (1969). *Medical records, medical education, and patient care.* Cleveland: Case Western Reserve University Press.

Werley, H., & Grier, M. (1981). *Nursing information systems.* New York: Springer.

Werley, H., & Lang, N. (Eds.). (1988). *Identification of the nursing minimum data set.* New York: Springer.

Zielstorff, R., Hudgings, C., & Grobe, S. (1993). *Next-generation nursing information systems: Essential characteristics for professional practice.* Washington, DC: ANA.

Zielstorff, R., McHugh, M., & Clinton, J. (1988). *Computer design criteria.* Kansas City, MO: ANA.

CHAPTER 6

Nurses' Changing and Emerging Roles with the Use of Unlicensed Assistive Personnel

Boni Johnson
Sally Friend
Julie MacDonald

Health care is undergoing dramatic change that challenges the nursing workforce to target their capabilities and resources. We assert that the time could not be more opportune or more critical for the redesign of health care roles in hospitals, beginning with registered nurses. This paper focuses on the new emerging RN roles that have resulted in the need for today's unlicensed assistive personnel (UAP).

Today a revolution is underway related to emerging roles for registered nurses. At the same time, there is much turmoil within the nursing profession related to job security and a sense of displacement from the job responsibilities that registered nurses have traditionally held.

Important to understanding the scope of emerging RN roles and the new accountabilities required is an exploration of the events that preceded the revolution. Many nurses saw themselves as victims or innocent bystanders to this movement of the mid-1990s. Nurses generally cite the proliferation of patient care redesign efforts as the precipitating event.

Hospital restructuring projects, often referred to as "patient-focused care," endeavored to serve patients better through decentralization and consolidation of care delivery and service providers. Continuity of care, bringing services closer to the patient, cross-training, and efficiency often were cornerstones of the redesign. One result often reported was a new addition to the patient care team known affectionately as unlicensed assistive personnel (UAP). This generic title was used most often because, although the specific job descriptions had some variability, their commonality lay in the fact that the individuals were not licensed and were used primarily in an assistive capacity to the registered nurse.

The resurgence of UAP roles may indeed have been a major precipitating event for a changing role for registered nurses. There are, however, more critical factors to be considered so that we can understand both the challenge and the opportunity in these emerging roles for nurses. Further, a different sequence of events may have actually occurred. It may have been the new emerging nursing roles, by design, that have resulted in the need for today's unlicensed, assistive personnel. The purpose of this chapter is to profile one hospital nursing department's journey redesigning the RN role and subsequently the role of the UAP. Emerging RN accountabilities, in light of a changing role and environment, will be explored. This chapter will challenge traditional thinking that patient care delivery can successfully be redesigned without first addressing the essential accountabilities within the role of the registered nurse.

BACKGROUND

Ferment and turmoil are not new to nursing, particularly within the hospital industry (Aiken, 1990, p. 72). Recurring cycles of nurse shortages and excess supply, coupled with the ongoing debate about how nurses should actually be spending their time are common themes (Prescott, Phillips, Ryan, & Thompson, 1991, p. 23). In the late 1980s, there were serious questions about whether nurses disliked the nursing shortage enough to cure it. Tough long-term strategies were posed, such as matching the role responsibilities of nurses and their salary according to their education and certification qualifications (Friss, 1988, p. 232). Nurse leaders implied that the shortage problem ought to be reframed from a shortage of nurses to a shortage of professional nursing. Long-term solutions present an ideal vision for the future but pose difficult implementation challenges given an existing workforce of nurses. Yet rapid change is occurring and heavily affecting nursing. Nurses either fear and retreat from change or embrace it as an opportunity to grow, develop, and strengthen professional nursing practice. Although dissatisfaction has been a common theme for nurses in hospital-based practice (Aiken, 1990, p. 78), fundamentally changing the role and adding focus and greater depth to new roles are not changes automatically embraced by RNs in practice. Change is unsettling and often threatening.

Lyon (1990) illuminated this issue and the difficulties inherent in the process by describing nursing work in *Getting Back on Track:*

> The adulteration of nursing and the resulting lack of consensus within the discipline on what we are about is our most serious and pressing, yet least attended to, problem. Lacking consensus, we lack unified direction in resolving our problems in both the educational and practice arenas. We get off track because we are not sure of what we are, and to compensate we try to be everything to everybody and pretend that all nurses have the same competencies in practice. Not having a clear and distinct identity, we often look like and feel like nobodies or, at best, substitutes for other health team members. By losing sight of who we are and what nursing is, we create an unnecessary sense of inadequacy and experience a paucity of pride in the discipline. Because we want more respect than we get and we want more status than we have, we often fight the wrong battles. (p. 267)

Lyon's message calls for consensus around nursing's essence coupled with subsequent action that keeps the discipline on track. This means fundamentally rethinking and critically analyzing the role of the RN.

For nurses at Lutheran Hospital in La Crosse, Wisconsin, this meant redefining nurse practice roles so that nurses embraced a common core definition of nursing and strengthened accountability for the full scope of nursing practice. Somehow, the full scope of nursing practice had become out of focus: As medicine had become increasingly more specialized over the past 15 years, nursing practice roles followed suit. This focus on the importance of medical specialization had detracted from the independent aspects of the RN's practice. Moreover, systems and social hierarchies were often developed within hospitals that recognized nurses in many ways for their willingness to adapt to these changes. For example, nurses at Lutheran Hospital in highly technical practice areas such as critical care received a greater share of benefits in enhanced shift differentials and educational allowances. Practices such as these caused dissension among nurses and gave the message that these highly technical skills were valued more than other skills that were prevalent on other patient care units, such as discharge planning, teaching, and counseling. Rediscovering nursing's common ground was a critical step in preparing for RN role redesign.

Although many definitions and theories of nursing had been influential in developing practice within Lutheran's nursing division, none seemed to provide the grounding being searched for as much as the work of Florence Nightingale did. Her simple descriptions of nursing as "the care that puts the patient in the best condition for nature to act" (Nightingale, 1859/1969, p. 133) and of health as "not only to be well but to be able to use well every power that we have" (Nightingale, 1893/1949, p. 6) became the basis for examining the processes within the essence of nursing. Nightingale's approach to both nursing and health called for a deeper knowing of each patient. Caring, knowing, empowerment, and facilitating the treatment that will put the patient in the best position for healing to occur became the foundation for nursing at Lutheran Hospital and the springboard for the role redesign that was to follow.

Lutheran Hospital's redesign efforts formally began in 1988, starting with the RN role as the focus for change. This change began with the recognition that a new consumer of health care was beginning to emerge. Further, economic factors were changing. Improving health status in a patient-focused environment required the renovation and restoration of professional nursing practice. With health, human response, and quality of life as new imperatives to be integrated into each individual's care, the way in which nursing care was organized and delivered clearly required a fundamental change.

To achieve the goals, RN roles were redesigned using a differentiated practice framework. The new framework essentially vested accountability for both the dependent and independent scopes of nursing practice. Two mutually valued roles were created: one role being more technical in nature, the other with a greater focus on health and human response. Together the two roles create a design for delivering the full scope of professional nursing practice. Moreover, nurses are more satisfied when their career aspirations and skills match role responsibilities that are assumed in ways that optimize their practice (American Association of Colleges of Nursing [AACN], 1995, p. 7). It is clear that as the social environment for nursing practice moves to a greater understanding of what really works best for each patient and as less emphasis is placed purely on tasks, nurses begin to appreciate what is unique about their contribution to patient care and what tasks are less critical for them to be actually doing themselves. Thus, delegation of tasks and differentiation of roles emerge and are valued.

Moreover, as patients and families have increased their roles as decision makers, as partners, and as providers, some of the control of nursing's traditional "doer" role has been displaced to the patients themselves and their support systems. What patients need at times is assistance, a coach, someone to help make judgments and help them evaluate the outcomes of care rather than a "rescuer" who takes over and creates dependency. This, too, is a real change in the emerging role of the nurse.

As nursing embraces its essence and then builds practice roles from that core essence, nurses begin to identify what makes a difference in care. Individual nurses still struggle with role identity and stress, however, while incorporating a new reality and changed work environment. Overall, the timing for RN role change could not have been better planned because the early to mid-1990s brought much turmoil and uncertainty in health care's external environment. RN role redesign not only centered nursing at the start of a new era in health care, it also paved the road for more change.

THE EVOLVING RESPONSE TO
TODAY'S CHANGING ENVIRONMENT

When nurses better understand patients and what makes a difference in their care, the work and the way in which it needs to be done fundamentally changes. This validates the redesigned RN roles and legitimizes a role for assistive personnel. When nurses gain depth in both understanding the health and human response of each patient and in the technical aspects of care, a two-fold opportunity arises. The first opportunity is to connect the patient with a team of care providers who will partner with the patient to achieve optimal wellness. The second opportunity evolves from the nurse's evaluation of the patient's response to interventions. Some outcomes will be predictable and routine; others may be unique and variable. This recognition allows the RN to assess the patient and determine those tasks that can be safely delegated and those that require further professional judgment and intervention by the nurse. Assistive personnel thus have a place as an integral part of the care delivery team.

Hospital staff feel they are being asked to do more with less. Confronting new issues with old solutions will not achieve needed improvements. New relationships with patients and among care providers are needed, and partnerships become the vehicle for accomplishing effective health care.

With shorter lengths of stay and an increased patient acuity during the hospital experience, time for the healing process is cut short. Time previously available for rest, meals, and family is often interrupted by frequent tests and treatments. In many instances, patients have received fragmented care from multiple services, resulting in redundancy and inefficiencies. Furthermore, brief incidental contacts by various staff who are often strangers to the patient occur in the performance of isolated functions. These conditions reflect an environment that has evolved rather than one that has been carefully designed around the needs of the patient. As professional nurses become more aware of the intrusive nature of illness and the specific affect on each patient, the obligation to design the conditions necessary for quality care and optimum healing becomes a major goal.

THE UAP BY DESIGN

According to DePree (1989), nurses need to develop a new concept of work—one that is productive, rewarding, meaningful, and fulfilling. Each worker has the right to be needed, to be involved, to understand, to have meaningful relationships, and to be accountable and contribute to the organization's goals. Employees need skills, discretion, incentives, and a structure that enables them to feel connected to the patient. Trust in the ability and intent of employees is a positive force in achieving patient-centered care. Valuing the contributions and differences of each care provider increases trust and produces the synergy desired among all team members. These principles apply directly to the differentiation of RN roles and the integration of the UAP into the care delivery team.

Restructuring care delivery requires a comprehensive approach because changing any one role affects all others. Clear and differentiated roles at Lutheran Hospital enhanced interdependence between nurses themselves and between nurses and UAP. Building a team that is responsible for the whole work process moves tasks closer to the patient and reduces the number of steps needed to complete tasks. Unlicensed assistive personnel, given training, support, and opportunity, can be effective team members fulfilling a needed role in the delivery of patient-centered care.

Unlicensed assistive personnel who are cross trained from a variety of different disciplines become multiskilled and are able to make a greater contribution to the work process. Positioning these care providers within the clinical team at the bedside places them in the stream for pertinent patient information and for delegation of assigned care by the RN. Moreover, being closer to the action and knowledgeable about what is actually going on with each patient supports better planning for the timing of each intervention, thus delivering services at hours more convenient and conducive to healing for the patient.

The outcome of redesign efforts at Lutheran Hospital resulted in the creation of an unlicensed assistant known as the patient care technician (PCT). These assistive personnel provide personal care for patients and perform unit activities to support and facilitate patient care. Additional training in a broad range of technical skills provides the PCT with the needed preparation to carry out appropriately delegated tasks, thus allowing the RNs to concentrate on those patient care responsibilities that only they can and should perform.

The design of the PCT role at Lutheran Hospital included those technical functions previously provided by centralized departments distant from the flow of information and patient activity. Patient contacts that had in the past been incidental were now incorporated into the PCT's routine care for the patient and into the patient's schedule. These new technical skills include phlebotomy and EKG. Expanded delegated tasks such as incentive spirometry, blood glucose monitoring, range of motion, and specimen collection assist with the implementation of the patient's prescribed plan of care. Observing and reporting the patient's response, status changes, and needs to the RN further supports and enhances the health care team and the patient's experience. Organizational and communication skills, confidentiality, and participation as a team member are standards expected of all Lutheran Hospital employees that round out the role of the PCT.

An effective approach to care redesign requires concomitant attention to the UAP role design and the new capabilities that are required of the registered nurse. A redesigned RN role, together with the complementary role of the UAP and the patient as a partner, creates a structure for delivering the aspired quality of care to the patient and family in the health care environment of today. Key to understanding the scope of the emerging RN role is the discovery and delineation of new qualifications that must be developed.

NEW ACCOUNTABILITIES FOR NURSES

What are the accountabilities now required of the RN as a new role emerges for the professional nurse? What new abilities must be integrated into the already vast storehouse of nursing knowledge? What functions will expand the scope of practice needed to take nursing into the future? Relational, reflective evaluation, care planning, and educational skills (see Table 6.1) make up the constellation of emerging RN role competencies needed for use with both patients and families as well as with UAP.

Relational Skills

With Patients and Families

First and foremost is the capacity to establish and sustain a relationship with the patient and family. The nurse needs to see the patient as a whole person and connect in a transforming way. Nurses need to be prepared to partner with patients and to care in new ways. This means establishing real and honest patient-nurse relationships and using mutuality (a balance of presenting one's

TABLE 6.1   Accountabilities for Nurses

Skill Area	RN Accountabilities	Emerging RN Accountabilities
Relational skills with patient and family	Follows customer service protocol	Establishes and sustains a partnership relationship
	Demonstrates competent performance of technical skill	Cares and creates healing space by spending nontask-related time with patient
Relational skills with UAP	Assumes a leadership role by coordinating the workshift	Uses time and skill to build trust and work collaboratively
Reflective evaluation skills with patient	Assesses current status data to select standards of care or nursing diagnosis	Understands and appreciates the patient's story/experience of health and illness as it affects their life (Tresolini, p. 30)
Reflective evaluation skills for self	Attends workshop in area of clinical expertise and shares information with colleagues	Learns through reflection on self and practice; uses an inquiry mode of learning (Tresolini, p. 26)
Care planning skills with patient and family	Establishes goals with patient and family	Encourages active collaboration of patient and family in choosing their own care
Care planning skills with UAP	Delegates aspects of care within shift according to education, expertise, and job description	Shares work responsibility in a mindful way
Educational skills with patient	Identifies and responds to learning needs	Informs patients of treatment choices and teaches self-care and responsibility for their own health
Educational skills with UAP	Orients UAP to role responsibilities	Mentors UAP

own thoughts and exploring others' thoughts) and self-disclosure for the purpose of developing relationships (Montgomery, 1993, pp. 43, 44).

Dialogue is a skill that enhances cooperation and identifies unique talents and coping mechanisms. The nurse adept at dialogue can encourage patients to experience and voice their vulnerabilities and emotions and to harness them for optimal health. Caring, involvement, and helping are expressed by spending nontask-related time with patients. This is a value-added aspect of the RN role that is underappreciated when time and tasks are focused on for efficiency reductions.

With Unlicensed Assistive Personnel

Relational skill is required in the emerging role of the RN, not only with the patient and family but with the unlicensed assistive personnel as well. Registered nurses need the ability to create trust with assistive personnel. This means that the RN knows what he or she is doing and can anticipate needs and be prompt. These RNs do what they say they will do and they follow through (Curtin, 1995, p. 8). They enjoy the work they have chosen to do. Time and skill are required to build trust, delegate, supervise, and work collaboratively with UAP.

The ability to delegate tasks and authority that do not require professional nursing expertise and training is essential for the nurse who is working with assistive personnel. The ability to share and negotiate the responsibility and authority is required (Gilmore, Hirschhorn, & O'Connor, 1994, p. 69). The RN must let go and let UAP do what they are capable of doing. The RN must allow assistive personnel the space to excel, yet manage accountability for patient care.

Today's nurses provide assistive personnel with resources and the rationale needed to accomplish the desired results. In newly emerging roles, they are available for advice, a pat on the back, the airing of ideas, or nonjudgmental discussion of differences. They take risks, live with dilemmas, and are willing to feel some discomfort as health care delivery moves toward increased integration.

These nurses convey a positive and caring professional image by believing in their own expertise and ability to make decisions. They have done their homework. They use respectful language. They take responsibility for their own actions and exercise choice. They dress for success and they laugh a lot! They celebrate accomplishments (Curtin, 1995, p. 8).

Reflective Evaluation Skills

With Patients and Families

A second ability necessary for the role of the RN is to reflect on their own thinking and reasoning—to use an inquiry mode of learning. Nurses make their own thinking visible to the patient and family and inquire into the patient's thinking and reasoning. Nurses value long-term thinking, use multiple sources of data to assess, diagnose, and plan care, and they embrace a systems thinking framework.

Professional judgment is used intuitively in relation to patients' unique needs and unique responses to nursing intervention. This nurse is not governed by conventional wisdom but is open to creativity and innovation and remembers that there are alternative viewpoints, goals, strategies, and processes. Diversity is appreciated and valued. Both intellect and emotion are embraced to enhance an understanding of situations and to create change. Disagreement is perceived as an opportunity to dig deeper.

These nurses are willing to take the risks required to change and grow. They are committed to lifelong learning of a body of nursing theory and technique; they have developed proficiency and expertise through practice. Common sense has not been abandoned.

With Unlicensed Assistive Personnel

Skilled competent care providers are integral to patient care. Assistive personnel need to be assured of the nurses' competence before they can trust enough to be connected to the team of health care providers. Assistive personnel have the right to be part of a competent team. The UAP need the opportunity to make a difference to the patient and family. They have the right to be held accountable for the work that they are hired to do.

Care Planning

With Patients and Families

When planning patient care, the nurse sees the patient beyond the work shift and this episode of illness. Thus, he or she can help the patient and family envision and design their future. Nurses advocate patient involvement in choosing their own care and honor the capacity of the patient, family, and other care providers to suggest alternatives to the plan of care.

Nurses come to understand what health, a health problem, or disability means to the patient and incorporate that knowing into the plan of care (AACN, 1995, p. 23). They ask the right questions and incorporate the patients' unique strengths and talents as well as resources for their problems into the plan of care. As they see opportunities for patient and family involvement in the doing, they help patients to help.

With Unlicensed Assistive Personnel

The registered nurse uses the patient care plan as a tool for giving UAP direction for their care activities. In this manner, both standard and individualized care is delivered by the health care team in a harmonious and comprehensive manner. Through the care plan, the assistive personnel can come to understand the patient's needs and the appropriate attentive response to those needs.

Education

For Patients and Families

These nurses understand the importance of giving information and explanations that patients can understand and use in their daily life. To encourage cost-conscious, meaningful choices that support the quality of life desired by the patient, nurses identify and teach what each patient needs to know. They inform patients about treatment alternatives and discuss how to monitor responses to that treatment. They teach the skills and tasks of caring for the self, thereby allowing patients to take responsibility for their own health.

For Unlicensed Assistive Personnel

Effective professional nurses teach the staff who assist them to make important decisions about organizing and conducting work activities. Nurses teach staff to plan and to carry out the work in ways that are most responsive to patient need.

Nurses personify and role-model the theory and concept of caring and have the ability to communicate a way of being present with the patient that allows the assistive personnel to care both for and about the patient. Relational communication skills are taught, so that the tasks performed by the unlicensed personnel are not perceived as dehumanizing, detached, or uncaring.

Nurses have the opportunity to teach new skills to UAP, thereby providing them with advancement opportunities, job security, and increased marketability. It is within the scope of the professional to both set and teach standards of care, practice, and performance.

Today's nurse must also be willing to learn from UAP. This humility involves being willing to let go of power over the assistant and being willing to be open and to trust the ability of the assistive staff. A learning environment is created where both learn from the other in an atmosphere of mutuality. A team spirit evolves creating energy and meaningful work as well as a healing space for the patient.

CONCLUSION

For many years the role of hospital registered nurses at the bedside has been one of evolution rather than one of careful design. Moreover, nursing in the past had positioned itself in a reactionary mode to changes in the environment, market, and the practice of other disciplines. Designing the role of nurses around accountabilities that flow from nursing's essence of caring, knowing, facilitating, and empowerment creates a necessary wholeness within the discipline and presents new opportunities to both deepen and expand the roles of registered nurses. Moving nursing from a ritual, task-based practice to one of critical understanding and reflection of what makes a difference for each patient changes both nursing's work and how care is delivered. The development of UAP in support of this design, and the values it represents, brings greater opportunity to center care specifically around the patient's needs and use the right person to do the right thing for each patient in the moment of care. New skills and abilities are required for nurses to serve the patient, the assistive personnel who are part of the team, the profession, and themselves with dignity and caring. This has been the proud tradition of nursing throughout its history.

REFERENCES

Aiken, L. H. (1990). Charting the future of hospital nursing. *Image: Journal of Nursing Scholarship, 22*, 72-78.

American Association of Colleges of Nursing, American Organization of Nurse Executives, and National Organization for Associate Degree Nursing. (1995). Monograph titled *A Model for Differentiated Nursing Practice.* Washington, DC: American Association of Colleges of Nursing.

Curtin, L. (1995). Management: Love it or leave it. *Nursing Management, 26*(6), 7-8.

DePree, M. (1989). *Leadership is an art.* New York: Bantam Doubleday Dell.

Friss, L. (1988). The nursing shortage: Do we dislike it enough to cure it? *Inquiry, 25*, 232-242.

Gilmore, T. N., Hirschhorn, L., & O'Connor, M. (1994, July-August). The boundaryless organization. *Healthcare Forum Journal*, 68-70.

Lyon, B. (1990). Getting back on track: Nursing's autonomous scope of practice. In N. Chaska (Ed.), *The nursing profession: Turning points* (pp. 267-274). St. Louis, MO: C. V. Mosby.

Montgomery, C. L. (1993). *Healing through communication.* Newbury Park, CA: Sage.

Nightingale, F. (1949). Sick nursing and health nursing. In I. Hampton (Ed.), *Nursing of the sick* (p. 6). New York: McGraw-Hill. (Original work published 1893)

Nightingale, F. (1969). *Notes on nursing.* New York: Dover. (Original work published 1859).

Prescott, P. A., Phillips, C. Y., Ryan, J. W., & Thompson, K. O. (1991). Changing how nurses spend their time. *Image: Journal of Nursing Scholarship, 23*, 23-28.

Tresolini, C. P., & Pew-Fetzer Task Force. (1994). *Health profession's education and relationship centered care.* San Francisco: Pew Health Professions Commission.

CHAPTER 7

Increasing Access to Health Care: The Indigenous Health Worker Option

Larry Anna Afifi

To provide effective, efficient health care to all clients has long been the aim of the health care professional. An increasing focus on cost containment and primary and preventive care is requiring health care providers not only to provide quality care but also to increase access to health care, increase use of available services, and improve patient outcomes. A major part of this clinic and outreach care effort involves using cultural beliefs, language, and methodology appropriate for the target community. One strategy for increasing access to and provision of effective and efficient care for diverse populations is the use of the indigenous health worker. The indigenous health worker can improve compliance and quality of care and access to care by providing selected programs and creating linkages between communities and health care settings. It is essential that the indigenous health worker program have community-based program planning, a well-defined training program, continuing education, adequate supervision, and program evaluation. A nurse manager is the ideal health professional to provide leadership for development and implementation of these activities.

By the year 2020, the population of the United States is estimated to increase to 325.9 million with various racial groups other than white totaling 22%. Between 1990 and 2020, the Asian American population will more than double its number (Kranczer, 1994). The Hispanic population is the fastest growing group in the United States and is expected to reach 21% of the population by the year 2050 (Rojas, 1994). By the year 2080, 51.1% of the population of the United States will be other than of white European background (Andrews, 1992). An obvious necessity, therefore, is that health professionals be conversant with multiple health belief systems and be able to provide culturally sensi- tive health care designed to meet the needs of specific populations (Witmer, Seifer, Finocchio, Leslie, & O'Neil, 1995).

Multiple determinants of health and health behavior have been identified throughout history. Cultural and social factors provide powerful determinants to health actions (Holmes, Hatch, & Robinson, 1992). The recognition of the major role of culture and environment in an individual's health and health behavior is critical to enable the health professional to diagnose and treat the health problem so that the individual will accept the treatment and comply. Concepts of illness and the role of the individual in various health and illness states vary greatly in different cultures (Basch, 1990). The health belief systems vary greatly, even among groups of white Americans.

Nurse roles have long included patient education, health promotion, and prevention activities. Standards of nursing care clearly state the necessity of providing care and education that is understood and accepted by the patient. On a daily basis, nurse managers are faced with providing care in acute and ambulatory care settings as well as outreach activities to individuals and groups with health beliefs, attitudes, and values toward health, illness, and death that differ from their own. Quality improvement programs require effective and efficient programs to meet identified needs of the target population. The dilemma, however, is how to reach these goals. How can programs be developed and implemented that meet the health needs of both health professionals and clients from diverse cultures? How can use of available services as well as compliance to medically sound preventive and treatment activities be improved? How can access to programs be improved? Above all, how can all this be accomplished within a cost containment climate?

CULTURALLY COMPETENT CARE

In this changing health world, it is critical to identify ways that can assist individuals to improve practices and conditions related to good health, assist in identifying resources that can increase the social support and decrease other stresses such as poverty and discrimination, and find a mediating capacity that can negotiate with professional agencies for better-quality services (Eng &

Young, 1992). Culturally competent nurses respect the unique culturally defined needs of each client individual or group and strive to provide services that reflect those needs (Roberts, 1990). The development of culturally sensitive programs denotes the ability of the health professional to understand the multiple determinants to health behavior. The acceptance is in practice that values and beliefs of cultures other than one's own are valid and appropriate for decision making, even if they differ from the nurse's own values and beliefs.

Perceived mutual respect and an understanding of cross-cultural communication and interaction styles between health professionals and lay persons are of primary importance for improved access, use, and program development for clients of different cultures (Malach & Segel, 1990). Health teaching in a cross-cultural setting requires more than a thorough knowledge of the subject matter (Harrison, 1992). Education is effective only if it can be internalized, and it can be internalized only if it is culturally relevant. Use of symbols and codes that are culturally specific enhance the native speaker's ability to portray the educational matter in several modes simultaneously, thus increasing the likelihood of comprehension. Role modeling and teaching strategies used by the health professional must use methods that best fit the intended target population.

What health care delivery systems are searching for is a method of providing culturally sensitive care to all individuals and communities. Although services may be available, inadequate use of the service is often an issue. Reasons for inadequate use are varied—lack of trust in the providers, perception of clients that available services do not understand their needs, and inability to explain their symptoms in English to professionals who support only the biomedical model, among others. Culture brokering is the process of "bridging gaps" between two systems, as between health professional and a cultural group (Jezewski, 1990). Nurses have been considered ideal culture brokers because their education stresses holistic care and patient advocacy. The additional use of the indigenous health worker operating as a team member with culturally competent nurses to provide cultural brokering may be one answer to the growing need for culturally relevant health care.

INDIGENOUS HEALTH WORKERS

There is no single accepted title for indigenous health care worker. They have been called community health workers, community health advisors, lay health workers, resource mothers, community health aides, health guides, peers, and many other names (Eng & Young, 1992; Giblin, 1989). The general role of this group of workers is described as nonprofessional members of the community who work to promote the health of individuals and communities. Generally, they work in communities that lack access or inadequately use available health care (Witmer et al., 1995). These health workers bridge gaps between the community and the health care system, helping the community understand the health care system (including its professionals) and helping the professionals understand the meanings of health and illness and the service needs from the client's point of view. Individuals of every culture frequently use their informal social support system to acquire help and information before they approach the formal health care system as well as during the illness process to verify their perceptions of the professional's advice (Melcher & Reichert, 1994). The indigenous health worker can act as that informal system as well as part of the formal health care system.

Indigenous health workers network with relevant cultures and provide services at the same time. These workers were first used in the United States in the 1950s when Native American health care workers were used to increase health care access for the Native American population (Melcher & Reichert, 1994). The Declaration of Alma-Ata (World Health Organization, 1978) identified community health workers as a major cornerstone in the ability of a nation to provide health care to all. The creation of culturally relevant programs through the use of a culturally competent professional staff working in cooperation with trained indigenous health workers relies heavily on the concept of a working team. Although it is impossible for any one nurse to understand cultural nuances, health beliefs, and attitudes of more than a few cultures, all nurses can be trained to be culturally competent. The roles of the nurse in these programs are multiple. Although at times the primary caregiver, the nurse will also be working in cooperation with the indigenous health worker on-site or at a distance. The nurse will often need to be the instigator of the program, working with other professionals and community members in the multiple roles of program designer, teacher, supervisor, and evaluator. All these roles require developing a trusting relationship between the indigenous health workers and the professional nurse. The creation of such a program is an ongoing collaborative process and requires that professional staff be comfortable with their knowledge and skills. They must also be able to share ownership and decision making with other professionals and individuals from the community (Roberts, 1990). Such programs should produce culturally relevant answers to some of our growing health problems.

Although many of the indigenous health worker programs in the United States and Canada are outreach programs, successful use of indigenous workers has been shown in a number of clinical programs. These include blood pressure screening, education, and follow-up in an emergency department (Bone et al., 1989), asthma education and follow-up (Butz et al., 1994), and diabetic control (Hopper, Miller, Birge, & Swift, 1984). Examples of outreach programs are those used for infant care (May, McLaughlin, & Penner, 1991; Poland, Giblin, Waller, & Bayer, 1991), children's health (Dawson, Cohrs, Eversole, Frankenburg, & Roth, 1976; Russo, Harvey, Kukafka, Supino, Freis, & Hamilton, 1982), health care for migrant families (Warrick, Wood, Meister, & de Zapien, 1992), HIV prevention (Freudenberg, 1990; Podschen, 1993), and cancer control (Michielutte, Sharp, Dengan, & Blinson, 1994).

Increasingly, the role of translator is being assigned to an indigenous health worker. Although family members are at times used as translators, cultural and social issues sometimes interfere with the direct translation of some health concerns or patient education. Medical translating requires more than just language skills. The translator must be able to understand the cultural beliefs and therefore discuss issues that may not have been raised (Haffner, 1992). It appears that the most ideal strategy to enhance client outcomes is the collaborative style of information transmission between the translator and the nurse (Hatton & Webb, 1993). Professional collaboration between the translator and the health professional needs to be developed through training and teamwork. When trusted indigenous workers provide education and information congruent with the advice of the health professional, the level of patient compliance is higher (Hatton & Webb, 1993; Holmes et al., 1992).

The indigenous health worker can be used in urban American settings to develop and implement a wide variety of programs, providing a mixture of curative and preventive services. Secondary to their training, nurses tend to give priority to medical solutions to health concerns, whereas the clients and the indigenous workers may give sociocultural or environmental factors priority. If both factors and solutions are not identified, compliance with medical solutions can be drastically reduced (Freudenberg, 1995; Jessee & Cecil, 1992). Development of nurse-indigenous health worker teams should allow a fuller understanding of these two aspects between the individual and the community.

The use of indigenous health workers increases the ability of health professionals to provide screening, expand program potential, provide culturally appropriate access to care that is identified as important by the community, identify barriers to care, target specific high-risk groups, and increase access to care. Indigenous workers provide outreach clinic tasks, offer health education, refer identified health problems to health professionals, obtain health histories, interpret health interviews and assessments, and generally act as change agents for the community and health service (Bray & Edwards, 1991; Butz et al., 1994;

Hopper et al., 1984). Cultural brokerage has been a relevant and recurrent theme (Mattson & Lew, 1992).

PROGRAM DEVELOPMENT

A number of issues have been identified as essential to make such programs work. First, the program development must be undertaken by a project team that includes health professionals and clients as well as influential others in the targeted community. The project team must include respected physicians and other health professionals in the specific health field being targeted (e.g., maternal-child health). Networking with the formal health community must be available at all levels during the program design and implementation. To provide for this, the program must bring into the planning phase, as well as into the advisory board, relevant members of the formal health community. Otherwise, access to the health system may be denied to the very clients you are trying to help. Warrick and associates (1992) noted that their program did not threaten the medical community, but it was also invisible to that community, possibly threatening the long-term sustainability of the program.

Community involvement in project design is essential (Swider & McElmurry, 1990). One barrier to indigenous worker programs can be resistance by professionals and bureaucratization of lay outreach programs. The development of an active community advisory board that includes key professionals may alleviate this problem.

Staff members must identify areas of personal concern that can hinder their ability to work with individuals from other cultures. Staff education about community values, beliefs, and concerns given by members of the targeted community as well as values clarification exercises are possible ways to approach this area. Roles for indigenous health workers are multiple and designed to fit the needs of each program. Each program must have an indigenous health worker job description to meet its needs.

According to the American Nurses Association (1994), an educational curriculum model of assessment, planning, implementation, and evaluation is essential for efficient and effective use of unlicensed assistive personnel (UAP). There are several critical components to the development of indigenous health worker programs (Table 7.1) (Butz et al., 1994; Giblin, 1989; Meister, Warrick, de Zapien, & Wood, 1992; Tiernan, 1988; Witmer et al., 1995).

Successful indigenous health worker programs take money and time to design and implement. Multiple benefits have been identified, however, for both the target group and the health services (Table 7.2) (Bone et al., 1989; Butz et al., 1994; Wells, DePue, Buehler, Lasater, & Carleton, 1990).

TABLE 7.1   Critical Components for Development of Indigenous Health Worker
Programs

1. Clear support and commitment from hospital or agency administration
2. Involvement of relevant and affected health professionals including physicians
3. Culturally relevant community involvement in developing, implementing, and evaluating
   programs
4. Selection of indigenous workers from the community
5. Acceptance by the target community
6. Staff training in cultural sensitivity and concepts of culturally competent services
7. Design of job descriptions and program procedures
8. Criterion-based training and continuing education of professional staff and indigenous
   health workers
9. Ongoing supervision and monitoring of indigenous workers and program elements
10. Strong evaluation components of all activities
11. Multiple interventions
12. Mutual trust and respect between professionals and indigenous health workers

TABLE 7. 2   Benefits of Indigenous Health Worker Programs

Target group perceives the indigenous health worker as

1. Able to explain the issue in everyday language
2. Able to understand barriers to health care and assisting them to overcome some of these
   barriers
3. Able to understand their needs
4. Credible sources of information
5. Positive role models

Health services views the indigenous worker as able to

1. Explain the community views to them
2. Provide culturally relevant information for identifying issues and problem-solving
3. Reach hard-to-reach populations with relevant information and programs
4. Assist in obtaining assessments and information for program design and evaluation
5. Know the cultural, environmental, and organizational factors in the community
6. Secure more immediate access to the community
7. Increase the health care provider's responsiveness and understanding of community needs
8. Act as a liaison between health professionals and the community, as individuals or groups
9. Provide support, both emotional and practical, that can improve client access to health
   care

SELECTION OF INDIGENOUS HEALTH WORKERS

Indigenous health workers are members of the target community. The target community may be multicultural, so the selection should be as close as possible to the cultural mix of the community. Melcher and Reichert (1994) suggested the importance of matching people based on shared attitudes. If no indigenous health worker is available from the same culture, it may be possible to match worker and client on the basis of other social attributes, such as immigrant status. The second aspect of the indigenous health worker position is assisting the health professional to understand the community. The worker must be able to interact with the health professional on a meaningful level. The selection process should be carefully designed before the first candidate is selected, with an evaluation component that allows changes in this process as needed.

EVALUATION OF EFFECTIVENESS

For each program, conscious identification of behavioral objectives with acceptable data levels for success must be identified during the program design. Effectiveness depends on prior ability to identify goals and objectives to be reached. Selected examples of such objectives are that an identified percentage of clients will be expected to comply with certain treatment guidelines, attend specified clinic activities, deliver normal birthweight babies, express satisfaction with the health program, or return to emergency rooms.

SUSTAINABILITY

The issue of sustainability of a program should be of major concern from the beginning of program design. Major outlays of time and expertise (translating into financial expense) are expended in initial design and implementation of any program. Methods of sustaining the program over time should be discussed before implementation.

Acceptability of the program goals and activities to both the professional and the targeted communities is essential for the continuation of any program. Involvement of these groups during program planning, implementation, and continuing evaluation helps ensure their continuing support. Accessibility pertains to both physical and psychological accessibility. The goals and location of the program must ensure physical access and psychological acceptability for the targeted populations.

The funding of any program is essential for long-term success. Even volunteer programs require funding for program design, training, supervision, and evaluation. The use of indigenous health workers does not identify whether or not these individuals are paid or volunteer. Swider and McElmurry (1990) referred to the need to provide salaries when indigenous health workers are poor women spending considerable amount of time on the project. Others have envisioned these programs as volunteer programs, with the payment being services, education, self-satisfaction, or other identified rewards (Hutchinson & Quartaro, 1993). If payment is not possible, there must be valued rewards built into the system to encourage extended participation by the indigenous health worker and provide program sustainability. One reason to use indigenous workers is to develop programs using available resources that enable a small budget to support a quality program. The use of nurse-indigenous worker teams allows improved access, quality care, and controlled budgets. Even if paid, indigenous workers will not require the same amount of money as professionals. The other argument is that to use volunteers from what is often the low-income population is not morally acceptable (Swider & McElmurry, 1990). The issue must be discussed for each program before implementation to improve sustainability.

INDIGENOUS HEALTH WORKERS IN
TUBERCULOSIS PREVENTION: A CASE EXAMPLE

Tuberculosis, although an "old" disease, is again a growing health concern in the world and in the United States. Although the entire population is at risk because tuberculosis is a silent airborne disease, several subgroups at highest risk are hard to reach, such as the homeless, HIV-positive individuals, and new immigrants from high-prevalence countries. Typically, urban areas have been hardest hit. New York City has successfully increased compliance in the active tuberculosis patient through a combined community-based organization using culturally concordant staff and providing related socioeconomic service programs in conjunction with direct observed therapy (DOT) workers (Klein & Naizby, 1995).

Freudenberg (1995) reported on the role of community organizations in the control of tuberculosis. Klein and Naizby (1995) reported on the use of community organizations in New York for mainly curative aspects of tuberculosis but also on the role community organizations can play in supporting the individual in social and environmental aspects. Cultural factors were identified as major reasons for failure to comply with active tuberculosis treatment in Quebec (Rideout & Menzies, 1994) and in Orange County (Rubel & Garro, 1992).

The Centers for Disease Control (1995) have urged the preventive treatment of high-risk groups with tuberculosis infection. Individuals newly arrived from high prevalence countries constitute one of these high-risk groups. At the University of Iowa, approximately 50% of all international students test positive for PPD and have negative chest X rays, thereby qualifying for preventive treatment. Although the preventive treatment program has been in place since 1987, very few students had taken part in the program. In the fall of 1992, an innovative program using indigenous health workers (peers) to assist in a two-prong attack for tuberculosis prevention therapy was initiated (McCue & Afifi, 1996). The program was developed after intensive discussions between Student Health Service (SHS), the Office of International Education and Services (OIES), various international student groups on campus, the County Public Health Department, and other interested faculty on campus. Although the program coordinator is a registered nurse and major program activity is undertaken by a second registered nurse, the involvement of physicians was essential for the sustainability of the program.

The program followed the recommended steps to success:

1. Community involvement in identifying the problem and solutions
2. Selection of peers from within the target population
3. Enthusiastic support of the program by the administration
4. Involvement in program design, training, and ongoing evaluation by relevant professional staff including state and county health department and SHS physicians
5. Job descriptions of lay health workers clearly identified
6. Competency-based training before activity and monthly continuing education
7. Ongoing supervision (weekly telephone calls, monthly meeting)
8. Available telephone contact from peer to immediate supervisor or program coordinator
9. Identified rewards for peers—cash payment not available
10. Training of SHS staff on cultural competence

Peers are used as cultural brokers between the professional staff and the clients. The professional staff uses the peer to assist in identifying international student concerns, discuss the meaning of screening results and reasons for isoniazid (INH) preventive therapy with students, assist in marketing preventive therapy to various international student groups, translate educational materials from English to a variety of languages, identify benefits and barriers of INH preventive therapy from the point of view of the international student, identify ways to increase compliance, and work directly with a specified number of students on preventive therapy. The peer provides the students with information in layman's terms, often in their own language; social, emotional, informational, and practical support as needed to facilitate INH preventive therapy compliance and to orient newcomers to the U.S. culture (including practical advice on where to buy ethnic groceries); and verification of their rights to refuse or comply.

After the introduction of this program, the compliance rate for INH preventive therapy increased from 5% to 79% during the first two years. SHS staff have become more culturally competent in dealing with international students during other clinic encounters as well. The improved compliance rate may be due to multiple factors: the improvement in staff cultural competence, improved international student understanding and therefore access to care, improved relationships with national student groups, a nurse assignment to the program on a regular basis, and direct contact by peers on a weekly basis. Although the peers are volunteers, the program requires both manpower and financial resources for sustainability. The improved compliance for tuberculosis prevention as well as improved access to care for other health care needs must be figured into the cost-benefit ratio, however.

CONCLUSION

At issue is the development of an attitude that allows an openness toward others' ideas of causation and treatment, with a clear understanding that there is rarely only one way to treat a health problem. If the lay solution is neutral or helpful, it should be considered along with the biomedical factors.

With the growing numbers of culturally diverse patients, an issue that has always been a concern for some health professionals (Leninger, 1978) has become a concern for all: the necessity to provide for culturally sensitive care at all levels of health care, from public health to emergency care (Andrews, 1992; Chalanda, 1995; D'Avanzo, 1992; Lea, 1994; Michielutte et al., 1994). The need to provide such care has led to the development of several innovative educational programs for students and continuing educational activities for professionals in the field. The recommendation to hire nursing staff from culturally diverse groups is valid. Unfortunately, it will be some time before the numbers of nurses from culturally diverse groups match the need. The profession of nursing is about caring. It is important that nurses learn to care for everyone and realize that biocultural definitions of health and illness vary widely. Even if a nurse is from, or intimately familiar with, a "minority" culture, he or she will not automatically understand the issues from all different cultures. Each health professional will interface with a variety of cultures within the health care setting. Even the use of the words *minority* or *underdeveloped nation* is offensive to those so designated. Who says an individual is a minority or a nation is underdeveloped?

To improve access to health care, nurses cannot afford *not* to use their expertise and training to move out of the hospital setting and into the communities from which their clientele come. This does not mean leaving hospital nursing but working together with epidemiologists, public health nurses, and others involved with health care to identify specific needs. Culturally competent nurses will be sensitive to the cultural issues and develop programs that are culturally relevant and acceptable to the targeted population (Jessee & Cecil, 1992). One method will be use of indigenous health workers. Indigenous health workers can improve compliance and quality of care as well as access to care by providing selected programs and creating linkages between communities and health care settings. It is essential for the indigenous health worker program to have community-based program planning, a well-defined training program, continuing education, adequate supervision, and program evaluation. A nurse manager is the ideal health professional to provide leadership for the development and implementation of these activities.

REFERENCES

American Nurses Association. (1994). *The registered nurse and the unlicensed assistive personnel (UAP)* (Brochure). New York: American Nurses Publishing.

Andrews, M. (1992). Cultural perspectives on nursing in the 21st century. *Journal of Professional Nursing, 8,* 7-15.

Basch, P. F. (1990). *Textbook of international health.* New York: Oxford Press.

Bone, L. R., Mamon, J., Levine, D. M., Walrath, J. M., Nanda, J., Gurley, H. T., Noji, E. K., & Ward, E. (1989). Emergency department detection and follow-up of high blood pressure. *American Journal of Emergency Medicine, 7,* 16-20.

Bray, M. L., & Edwards, L. H. (1991). Prevalence of hypertension among Hispanic Americans. *Public Health Nursing, 8,* 276-280.

Butz, A.M., Malveaux, F. J., Eggleston, P., Thompson, L., Schneider, S., Weeks, K., Huss, K., Murigande, C., & Rand, C. S. (1994). Use of community health workers with inner-city children who have asthma. *Clinical Pediatrics, 33,* 135-141.

Centers for Disease Control and Prevention. (1995). Essential components of a tuberculosis prevention and control program and screening for tuberculosis and tuberculosis infection in high-risk populations: Recommendations of the Advisory Council for the Elimination of Tuberculosis. *Morbidity and Mortality Weekly Review, 44*(No. RR-11), 1-33.

Chalanda, M. (1995). Brokerage in multicultural nursing. *International Nursing Review, 42,* 19-22.

D'Avanzo, C. E. (1992). Barriers to health care for Vietnamese refugees. *Journal of Professional Nursing, 8,* 245-253.

Dawson, P., Cohrs, M., Eversole, C., Frankenburg, W., & Roth, M. (1976). Cost-effectiveness of screening children in housing projects. *American Journal of Public Health, 66,* 1192-1194.

Eng, E., & Young, R. (1992). Lay health advisors as community change agents. *Family and Community Health, 15,* 24-40.

Freudenberg, N. (1990). AIDS prevention in the United States: Lessons from the first decade. *International Journal of Health Services, 20,* 589-599.

Freudenberg, N. (1995). A new role for community organizations in the prevention and control of tuberculosis. *Journal of Community Health, 20,* 15-28.

Giblin, P. T. (1989). Effective utilization and evaluation of indigenous health care workers. *Public Health Reports, 104,* 361-368.

Haffner, L. (1992). Translating is not enough: Interpreting in a medical setting. *Western Journal of Medicine, 157,* 255-259.

Harrison, M. (1992). Towards effective intercultural teaching. *Nursing Administration Quarterly, 16,* 29-34.

Hatton, D. C., & Webb, T. (1993). Information transmission in bilingual, bicultural contexts: A field study of community health nurses and interpreters. *Journal of Community Health Nursing, 10,* 137-147.

Holmes, A., Hatch, J., & Robinson, G. (1992). A lay educator approach to sickle cell disease education. *Journal of National Black Nurses Association, 5*(2), 26-38.

Hopper, S. V., Miller, P., Birge, C., & Swift, J. (1984). A randomized study of the impact of home health aids on diabetic control and utilization patterns. *American Journal of Public Health, 74,* 600-602.

Hutchinson, R. R., & Quartaro, E. G. (1993). Training imperatives for volunteers caring for high-risk, vulnerable populations. *Journal of Community Health Nursing, 10,* 87-96.

Jessee, P. O., & Cecil, C. E. (1992). Evaluation of social problem-solving abilities in rural home health visitors and visiting nurses. *Maternal-Child Nursing Journal, 20,* 53-64.

Jezewski, M. A. (1990). Culture brokering in migrant farmworker health care. *Western Journal of Nursing Research, 12,* 497-513.

Klein, S., & Naizby, B. (1995). New linkages for tuberculosis prevention and control in New York City: Innovative use of nontraditional providers to enhance completion of therapy. *Journal of Community Health, 20,* 5-13.

Kranczer, S. (1994). Outlook for U. S. population growth. *Statistical Bulletin—Metropolitan Insurance Companies, 75,* 19-26.

Lea, A. (1994). Nursing in today's multicultural society: A transcultural perspective. *Journal of Advanced Nursing, 20,* 307-313.

Leninger, M. (1978). Transcultural nursing theories and research approaches. In M. Leninger (Ed.), *Transcultural Nursing* (pp. 31-51). New York, John Wiley.

Malach, R. S., & Segel, N. (1990). Perspectives on health care delivery systems for American Indian families. *Child Health Care, 19,* 219-228.

Mattson, S., & Lew, L. (1992). Culturally sensitive prenatal care for Southeast Asians. *Journal of Obstetric, Gynecologic, and Neonatal Nursing (JOGNN), 21,* 48-54.

May, K. M., McLaughlin, F., & Penner, M. (1991). Preventing low birth weight: Marketing and volunteer outreach. *Public Health Nursing, 9,* 97-104.

McCue, M., & Afifi, L. A. (1996). Using peer helpers for tuberculosis prevention. *Journal of American College Health, 44,* 173-176.

Meister, J. S., Warrick, L. H., de Zapien, J. G., & Wood, A. H. (1992). Using lay health workers: Case study of a community-based prenatal intervention. *Journal of Community Health, 17,* 37-51.

Melcher, C., & Reichert, T. (1994, November). Lay health advisors: A critique and analysis of the field. Paper presented at Eightieth Annual Meeting of Speech Communication Association, New Orleans.

Michielutte, R., Sharp, P., Dengan, M., & Blinson, K. (1994). Cultural issues in the development of cancer control programs for American Indian populations. *Journal of Health Care for the Poor and Underserved, 5,* 280-296.

Podschen, G. (1993). Teen peer outreach-street work project: HIV prevention education for runaway and homeless youth. *Public Health Reports, 108,* 150-155.

Poland, M. L., Giblin, P. T., Waller, J. B., & Bayer, I. S. (1991). Development of a paraprofessional home visiting program for low-income mothers and infants. *American Journal of Preventive Medicine, 7*, 204-207.

Rideout, M., & Menzies, R. (1994). Factors affecting compliance with preventive treatment for tuberculosis at Mistassini Lake, Quebec, Canada. *Clinical Investigative Medicine, 17*, 31-36.

Roberts, R. N. (Ed.). (1990). Developing culturally competent programs for children with special needs. (Monograph and workbook). Washington, DC: Georgetown University Child Development Center.

Rojas, D. (1994). A case in role development. *Nursing and Health Care, 15*, 258-261.

Rubel, A. J., & Garro, L. C. (1992). Social and cultural factors in the successful control of tuberculosis. *Public Health Reports, 107*, 626-636.

Russo, R., Harvey, B., Kukafka, R., Supino, P., Freis, P., & Hamilton, P. (1982). The use of community health aides in a school health program. *Journal of School Health, 52*, 425-427.

Swider, S. M., & McElmurry, B. J. (1990). A women's health perspective in primary health care: A nursing and community health worker demonstration project in urban America. *Family and Community Health, 13*(3), 1-17.

Tiernan, K. M. (1988). Training volunteers in risk-reduction education: A program in a U.S.-Mexican border community. *Family and Community Health, 11*, 60-72.

Warrick, L., Wood, A., Meister, J., & de Zapien, J. (1992). Evaluation of a peer health worker prenatal outreach and education program for Hispanic farmworkers' families. *Journal of Community Health, 17*, 13-26.

Wells, B. L., DePue, J. D., Buehler, C. J., Lasater, T. M., & Carleton, R. A. (1990). Characteristics of volunteers who deliver health education and promotion: A comparison with organization members and program participants. *Health Education Quarterly, 17*, 23-25.

Witmer, A., Seifer, S. D., Finocchio, L., Leslie, J., & O'Neil, E. H. (1995). Community health workers: Integral members of the health care work force. *American Journal of Public Health, 85*, 1055-1058.

World Health Organization. (1978). *Alma-Ata 1978: Primary Health Care.* Geneva: World Health Organization.

CHAPTER 8

Life Care Nursing Management in Long-Term Care

Jeanette M. Daly

Exciting changes are occurring in health care impacting on long-term care delivery systems. At the national level lawmakers are negotiating reforms that will change the way providers do business. This affects the acuity level of residents and is changing the services provided in long-term care. At one end of the spectrum is the assisted living services and at the other end are the special care units. This chapter discusses the changing health care delivery environment in long-term care and describes a model of life-care management used in a midwestern life-care home. Specific aspects of this model are discussed including the philosophy, nursing delivery mode, organizational structure, role descriptions, staffing patterns, and a description of the interdisciplinary health care team. Evaluation of the life-care management model described in this chapter is supported by patient outcomes, nursing turnover, calculations, and the results of a nursing job satisfaction survey.

It may at first appear paradoxical to name a nursing home's nursing model "life care." As the geriatric population both grows in numbers and lives longer, however, "life care" appropriately speaks to the continuity of nursing services in long-term care settings. Registered nurses (RNs) play a key role in the continually changing long-term care environment. The RNs are at the heart of the life care nursing model.

Oaknoll Retirement Residence is a nonprofit life care home that provides nursing services for persons residing independently in apartments or living in the health center on a temporary or permanent basis. As a long-term care facility, the impact of health care reform remains on the minds of administration and nursing. New systems will continue to emerge in the health care environment. As a long-term care facility, Oaknoll must be progressive and willing to work within a changing health care environment.

In this chapter, I will discuss the changing health care environment in long-term care and the inherent changes for Oaknoll. The life care nursing model will be described along with Oaknoll's philosophy, organizational structure, and description of the interdisciplinary health care team. Evaluation of the model will be supported by organizational and patient outcomes. Organizational outcomes include nursing turnover indices and survey results for facility relicensure. Patient outcomes consist of care plan analysis and patient use of psychoactive medications, physical restraints, and indwelling catheters and presence of pressure sores.

HEALTH CARE DELIVERY ENVIRONMENT
IN LONG-TERM CARE

Exciting changes are occurring in health care. The changes are affecting long-term care delivery systems. At a national level, lawmakers are negotiating reforms that will change the way providers do business. New guidelines on the acuity level of the residents will add more services to long-term care. At one end of the spectrum are assisted living services, and at the other end are subacute care units (Wallach, 1994). With our life care philosophy, Oaknoll must position itself to provide the continuum of services for its residents, from independent living, to assisted living, to special care in either a skilled or intermediate care setting.

O'Connor (1994) noted the fast pace of nursing facilities refocusing and expanding their health care delivery efforts. Many more nursing facilities are offering assisted living, special care units, and home care services. The typical nursing facility offering just one service of long-term care will not be able to survive in the future and will need to expand with a variety of services. Oaknoll, with a life care philosophy, has established a variety of services. If an apartment resident requires rehabilitation, it is provided. If an apartment resident has a tracheotomy and needs skilled nursing care, that also is provided. Those services that residents need will be available. This concept differs from those who specialize in subacute care.

Subacute care is "comprehensive inpatient care designed for someone who has an acute illness, injury, or exacerbation of a disease process. It is goal-oriented treatment rendered immediately after, or instead of, acute hospitalization to treat one or more specific active complex medical conditions or to administer one or more technically complex treatments, in the context of a person's underlying long-term conditions and overall situation" ("AHCA, JCAHO," 1994, p. 9). Oaknoll must provide a variety of health care services that do not cluster into a bundle that lends itself to the formation of a specific subacute care unit.

MODES OF NURSING CARE DELIVERY

The mode of delivery of nursing care can vary from institution to institution. Differences can also be found within a facility from unit to unit and evolve over time. The earliest form of nursing care was the "case method" of delivery. This method allowed the nurse to provide care on a one-to-one basis. In a sense, primary nursing is similar to case method nursing, one nurse is assigned to each patient. But as Marram, Barrett, and Bevis (1979) noted in primary nursing, the nurse assigned to each patient is responsible for 24 hours a day until the patient is discharged. A difference from the case method is noted with primary care in that after one's shift of duty the responsibility for the patient is transferred to the oncoming nurse. At Oaknoll, nursing care is similar to both of those methods (Lee, 1993).

Life care nursing goes beyond primary or case method philosophies and takes on a case management approach. As is evident in the literature, there are many approaches to case management and just as many definitions. "Case management may describe a patient care delivery system, a professional practice model, a group of activities that a nurse performs within an organizational setting, or a separate service provided by private practitioners" (Goodwin, 1994, p. 29). The scope of case management at Oaknoll is broader than usual because of the continuum of independent to dependent living situations. Zander (1990) differentiated case management while focusing on a provider continuity with managed care. She defined managed care as "a clinical system for the strategic management of cost and quality outcomes" (Zander, 1990, p. 1) and stated that both continuity of care and provider is necessary for quality outcomes. Geron and Chassler offered a long-term care definition for case management: "a service that links and coordinates assistance from both paid service providers and unpaid help from family and friends to enable consumers with chronic functional and/or cognitive limitations to obtain the highest level of independence consistent with their capacity and their preferences for care" (1994, p. v).

Case management at Oaknoll is closer to Geron and Chassler's definition, which lends itself to chronic disabilities of the elderly. Nursing at Oaknoll also corresponds to the ANA definition of case management as "a system with many elements: health assessment, planning, procurement, delivery and coordination of services, and monitoring to assure that the multiple service needs of the client are met" (American Nurses Association, 1988, p. 1).

OAKNOLL'S LIFE CARE NURSING MODEL

Nursing care at Oaknoll is provided by registered nurses, licensed practical nurses, and certified nurse assistants. The philosophy of a life care home is that health care needs will be met for life after entry into the system. Residents will receive health care services in a cost-effective, quality manner. Oaknoll has 133 apartments for persons in independent living and a 48-bed health center for persons either temporarily or permanently ill. The health center is licensed to provide skilled and intermediate levels of care (Graham et al., 1987). Set criteria have been established for admission to Oaknoll in the independent area. Future residents must be 65 years or older, in good health, and meet financial requirements.

Entry into the life care home in independent living initiates a visit from nursing. Many new residents at Oaknoll do not need nursing care. They are independent in living situations. They are introduced to nursing when first moving into Oaknoll through the "Vial of Life," a questionnaire that asks for vital health information from the new resident. If information is not available, such as a physician name or a list of current medications, nursing collaborates with the resident to complete the information. Meetings held by floor in the independent living complexes are also provided to introduce and clarify nursing services that are provided for persons in independent living. An independent living resident can call on nursing through different referral mechanisms; for example, a crisis such as a fall and fractured hip, administrator's concern about loss of weight, apartment resident's concern about requests to cook another resident's meals, another nonnursing Oaknoll employee's concern that a resident sleeps all day, family's concern that resident's hygiene is no longer adequate, nurse's concern that short-term memory is impaired, patient's concern that gait is unsteady, physician's concern that medications are not being taken as prescribed, and significant other's concern that apartment is unkempt and not safe. Usually one or more of the following lead to either a temporary or permanent admission to the health center: a chronic illness or catastrophic event, history of frequent hospital or nursing facility admissions, inadequate caregiver, cognitive deficit, or emotional support/deficit. Figure 8.1 depicts Oaknoll's Life Care Model that comprises two interrelated components (Gibbs, Lonowski, Meyer, & Newlin, 1995), which are the nursing process offered in two settings: the health center or apartments.

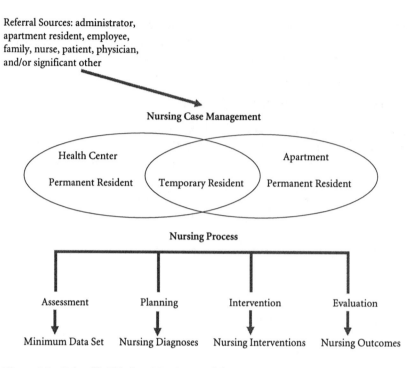

Referral Sources: administrator,
apartment resident, employee,
family, nurse, patient, physician,
and/or significant other

Nursing Case Management

Health Center   Apartment

Permanent Resident   Temporary Resident   Permanent Resident

Nursing Process

Assessment   Planning   Intervention   Evaluation

Minimum Data Set   Nursing Diagnoses   Nursing Interventions   Nursing Outcomes

Figure 8.1: Oaknoll's Life Care Nursing Model

After a resident is admitted by a physician order, a registered nurse is assigned primary responsibility for this client by the director of nursing (DON). This nurse is responsible for the assessment, planning, implementation, and evaluation of the resident's care for life. This primary responsibility for patient care has been ongoing since 1990 and is a new role for nurses at Oaknoll. As mandated by the Omnibus Reconciliation Act 1987 (OBRA), in long-term care a minimum set of data (MDS) must be collected as the initial assessment used by nurses to collect information about a patient. After completion of the MDS, 18 different areas can be triggered on the resident assessment instrument (RAPS) (e.g., delirium, cognitive loss, communication, ADL [activities of daily living] functional, visual function, urinary incontinence, etc.) (Federal Register, 1991). These areas are reviewed by the primary nurse, and then nursing diagnoses are formulated and a care plan developed to meet the identified needs (Bolander, 1994).

Nursing in a life care facility, like case method care and primary nursing, assigns one nurse to each patient. That nurse is responsible for the patient 24 hours a day for the duration of the patient's stay at Oaknoll. Together with the resident and interdisciplinary health care team, the nurse formulates and implements the plan of care. Not all interventions planned are implemented by the nurse because many of the duties are delegated to other health center personnel. Currently, the 11 nurses responsible for residents' care have been employed at Oaknoll for more than 5 years.

As the Life Care Model depicts, the primary nurse implements the nursing process for the resident while in the health center but also if the resident is discharged to his or her apartment. The nurse continues responsibilities for this client. Residents needing nursing care in their apartments have a variety of services available to them including companions, meals, medication and treatments, life line for emergency calls for help, and peer counseling. If a specific problem occurs for residents once they are back in their apartments, the primary nurse is consulted for interventions. This role of the primary nurse facilitating a resident's care after discharge from the health center is an evolving role.

Interdisciplinary Health Care Team

Nursing is one discipline involved in the interdisciplinary health care team at this facility. The resident's primary nurse, director of nursing, nurse assistant, and rehabilitation aide attend the resident's care plan conference. Other involved team members are supervisors from the dietary and activity departments, along with the physician, patient, family or significant other, and consultants from the areas of social work, dietary, physical therapy, occupational therapy, and speech therapy.

The consulting social worker is responsible for coordinating the weekly care plan conferences. The social worker invites the resident, family, and physician and coordinates scheduling all other disciplines to attend the meetings. Each conference is led by the resident's nurse who reviews each patient problem. Under the auspices of the nursing process, goals, and interventions are identified and the care plan team works together sharing ideas to meet the needs and solve the problems of the residents. Residents and their families are active members in this process when possible.

Care plans at Oaknoll became computerized in 1992, and change has occurred in the structure of the care plan. Standardized nursing language is used for two components of the nursing process. North American Nursing Diagnosis Association (NANDA) nursing diagnoses are used for the patient's problem statements and interventions from Nursing Interventions Classification (NIC) are used as approaches or orders that nurses carry out (Iowa Intervention Project, 1992; NANDA, 1994). The process of health care and nursing model have been described and evaluation of the outcomes will be discussed.

TABLE 8.1   Number and Percent of Patient Outcome by Year at Oaknoll.

Outcomes	1991 N = 38	1992 N = 38	1993 N = 34	1994 N = 39
Pressure Sores	1 (3%)	2 (5%)	0	1 (3%)
Psychoactive Medication Use	5 (9%)	2 (5%)	1 (3%)	5 (13%)
Indwelling Catheter	2 (5%)	2 (5%)	2 (6%)	2 (5%)
Physical Restraint Use	2 (5%)	1 (3%)	0	1 (3%)

Evaluation

Formal evaluation of the life care nursing model at Oaknoll has not been completed as an entity by itself but will be addressed by organizational and patient outcomes. Kane (1995) noted that improving the quality of long-term care can be measured with outcomes. Patient outcomes as required by state audits for nursing facility relicensure were chosen for presentation. These include use of psychoactive medication, use of indwelling catheters, use of physical restraints, and prevalence of pressure sores. In addition, the number and frequency of use of nursing diagnoses and interventions are presented. Organizational outcomes presented are nursing turnover indices and state survey for relicensure results. Turnover is the number of employees who voluntarily or involuntarily leave their jobs during a year. Indices include crude turnover rate, survival rate, and wastage rate (see Appendix A for turnover indices calculations and definitions) (Duxbury & Armstrong, 1982; Hofmann, 1981).

Patient outcomes are provided by year at the time Oaknoll had the annual survey for relicensure. The list of patient outcomes are those required for survey information for relicensure and examples are indwelling catheter use, incidence of pressure sores, psychoactive medication use, and physical restraint use. Categories are set by the Department of Health and Human Services rules and regulations. Table 8.1 lists the census number and patient outcomes for health center residents from 1991 to 1994.

Restraint use, incidence of pressure sores, catheter use, and psychoactive medication use is low at Oaknoll compared with the norms in long-term care. In skilled and nursing home-type facilities, the prevalence of pressure ulcers for residents was discovered to be 23% (Langemo, Olson, Hunter, Burd, Hansen, & Cathcart-Silberberg, 1989; Young, 1989). A pressure sore of only 3% in 1994 and 5% in 1992 is tremendous compared with prevalence rates ranging from 2.6% to 24% (Brandeis, 1990). Also restraint reduction promoted through OBRA 1987 is evident at Oaknoll with a range of 3% to 5% in the years

TABLE 8.2. Number and Frequency of Nursing Diagnoses and Interventions Use
for Eight Time Periods for Care Plans of Residents in Health Center.

	2/91	8/91	2/92	8/92	3/93	8/93	2/94	8/94
Census	42	39	41	28	35	33	40	36
Number of Nursing Diagnoses	30	30	49	38	44	44	44	45
Frequencies of Nursing Diagnoses	185	172	256	203	255	309	345	316
Mean N Dx/Care Plan	4.4	4.4	6.2	7.2	7.3	9.4	8.6	8.7
Number of Nursing Interventions	0	0	0	95	107	110	121	111
Frequencies of Nursing Interventions	0	0	0	445	503	584	671	598
Mean N Int/Care Plan				15.9	14.3	17.7	16.8	16.6

reported on. Nationally, in 1989 after OBRA 1987, 41% of all nursing home
residents were placed in restraints (Tinetti, Liu, & Ginter, 1992). Mahoney
(1995) affirmed the number of residents restrained at 37%.

Computerized care plans were available in August 1991. At that time, the
NIC interventions were initiated for care plan use. Before this, only the NANDA
nursing diagnoses were used as a standardized language at Oaknoll. Since the
inception of computerization and the standardized languages, care plans have
changed and now include many more nursing diagnoses and interventions. See
Table 8.2 for frequency of use of nursing diagnoses and interventions.

Turnover indices have been calculated for the same years presented for
patient outcomes. Figures for nurses and nurse assistants are presented in Table
8.3. The annual nurse crude turnover rates are low-ranging from 13.9% to
18.7%. This is exceptional and much lower than the national reportings for
nurse turnover in long-term care at 45.8% (Crowley, 1993). The nurse assistant
crude turnover rate at Oaknoll was, not surprisingly, higher than that of the
nurses and ranged from 62% to 87.5%. The nurse assistant crude turnover is
one of the major problems of the long-term care industry and McDonald
(1994) reported a national average of 50% turnover for nurses assistants that
ballooned as high as 400% in some facilities. In 1992, Crowley (1993) reported
the national nurse assistant turnover was 80.1%. Waxman, Carner, and
Berkenstock (1984) noted that organizational effectiveness is problematic
when turnover exceeds 50%. At Oaknoll, crude turnover has progressively
decreased in percentage and for two years has stayed in the lower 60%.

From the results of survival and wastage rates for the nursing staff, more than
half of the newly hired employees remained in their jobs during a 12-month
period. New employees, both nurses and nurse assistants, who left in each year
still seem to constitute a large percentage of former employees, however.

TABLE 8.3   Turnover and Survival Rates for Nurses and Nurse Assistants for Four
Years (in percentages).

	Nurses			Nurse Assistants		
	Crude	Survival	Wastage	Crude	Survival	Wastage
1994	13.9	66	34	60	65	35
1993	14.6	100	0	62	69	31
1992	16.2	50	50	93	51	49
1991	18.7	80	20	87.5	60	40

TABLE 8.4   List of Deficiency Citations for Four Years at Oaknoll

1991 Survey Results:
   Nutritional needs were not met
   Nutritional substitutes were not offered
   All employees were not trained in emergency procedures
   Resident rights were not given yearly
   Survey results were not posted

1992 Survey Results:
   Adequate dining room space was not provided
   No ongoing activities program existed
   Staff failed to assist persons to eat in a timely manner

1993 Survey Results:
   No deficiencies

1994 Survey Results:
   No deficiencies

Patient outcomes and turnover indices provided employee and patient information and survey citation data provide an overall organizational picture of what was occurring at Oaknoll. Table 8.4 provides a list of survey results for four years with detail of deficiency citations. Over time, deficiency citations have decreased at Oaknoll. The state norm for 1994 was an average of 8 deficiencies per long-term care facility. Oaknoll was below that average for each of the years discussed.

SUMMARY

Evaluation of nursing at this life care home reveals that quality is the result of hard work and effort. The primary nurses with the interdisciplinary care plan team have improved each resident's care plan, which has resulted in more personalized care with all needs identified. As shown by improved patient outcomes, increased use of nursing diagnoses and interventions, low nurse turnover rate, and decreased deficiency citations during state relicensure process, the nursing care at Oaknoll is excellent. This outcome was achieved by the vision and guidance of nursing administration coupled with improvement efforts spearheaded by nursing. The life care nursing model reflects nurses' values and knowledge joined by a commitment to continuous care improvement and the development of a nursing system that focuses on patients. It is difficult to identify what specifically accounts for these positive outcomes, but certainly the nursing model as described has an definite influence.

A deep personal and professional commitment from each and every employee in each and every department is needed to achieve quality care. "Quality is a continuous journey of awareness, performance and evaluation" (Molloy, 1994, p. 36). It is fortunate that the director of nursing at Oaknoll has advanced education with a focus in nursing administration. Knowledge of management, organization theory, finance, marketing and planning, personnel administration, supervision, and nursing is a necessity for DONs in long-term care (Ballard, 1995). Oaknoll's DON has this background and has influenced the direction of nursing in this life care home.

REFERENCES

AHCA, JCAHO endorse subacute care definition. (1994). *Provider, 20*(10), 8-9.

American Nurses Association. (1988). *Nursing case management.* Publication No. NS-32. Kansas City, MO: American Nurses Association.

Ballard, T. M. (1995). The need for well-prepared nurse administrators in long-term care. *Image: Journal of Nursing Scholarship, 27*(2), 153-154.

Bolander, V. R. (1994). *Basic nursing: A psychophysiologic approach.* Philadelphia: W. B. Saunders.

Brandeis, G. (1990). The epidemiology and natural history of pressure ulcers in elderly nursing home residents. *Journal of the American Medical Association, 264*, 2905-2909.

Crowley, C. H. (1993). The human factor: Unmasking staff potential. *Provider, 19*(12), 22-32.

Duxbury, M. L., & Armstrong, G. D. (1982). Calculating nurse turnover indices. *The Journal of Nursing Administration, 12*, 18-24.

Federal Register. (1991, September 26). Medicare and Medicaid: Requirements for long-term care facilities and nurse aide training and competency evaluation programs, final rules. Washington, DC: Department of Health and Human Services, 48826-48922.

Geron, S. M., Quinn, J. (1994). *Guidelines for case management practice across the long-term care continuum.* Bristol, CT: Connecticut Community Care.

Gibbs, B., Lonowski, L., Meyer, P. J., & Newlin, P. J. (1995). The role of the clinical nurse specialist and the nurse manager in case management. *Journal of Nursing Administration, 25*(5), 28-34.

Gold, M. F. (1993). Reflection on the future. *Provider, 19*(12), 39-40.

Goodwin, D. R. (1994). Nursing case management activities: How they differ between employment setting. *Journal of Nursing Administration, 24*(2), 29-34.

Graham, P., Constantini, S., Balik, B., Bedore, B., Hooke, M. C. M., Papin, D., Quamme, M., & Rivard, R. (1987). Operationalizing a nursing philosophy. *Journal of Nursing Administration, 17*(3), 14-18.

Hofmann, P. B. (1981). Accurate measurement of nursing turnover: The first step in its reduction. *The Journal of Nursing Administration, 11*, 37-39.

Iowa Intervention Project. (1992). *Nursing Interventions Classification (NIC)*. St. Louis, MO: Mosby-Year Book.

Kane, R. L. (1995). Improving the quality of long-term care. *Journal of the American Medical Association, 273*(17), 1376-1380.

Langemo, D. K., Olson, B., Hunter, S., Burd, C., Hansen, D., & Cathcart-Silberberg, T. (1989). Incidence of pressure sores in acute care, rehabilitation, extended care, home health, and hospice on one locale. *Decubitus, 2*(2), 42.

Lee, J. L. (1993). A history of care modalities in nursing. *Series on Nursing Administration, 5*, 20-38.

Mahoney, D. F. (1995). Analysis of restraint-free nursing homes. *Image: Journal of Nursing Scholarship, 27*(2), 155-160.

Marram, G., Barrett, M. W., & Bevis, E. O. (1979). *Primary nursing*. St. Louis, MO: C. V. Mosby.

McDonald, C. A. (1994). Recruitment, retention, and recognition of frontline workers in long-term care. *Generations, XVIII*(3), 41-42.

Molloy, G. E. (1994). Quality is the administrator's job #1. *Nursing Homes, 43*(8), 36-39.

North American Nursing Diagnosis Association (1994). *NANDA nursing diagnoses: Definitions and classification 1995-1996*. Philadelphia: North American Nursing Diagnosis Association.

O'Connor, J. (1994). Facilities diversity to meet future demand. *McKnight's Long-Term Care News, 15*(7), 3.

Tinetti, M., Liu, W., & Ginter, S. F. (1992). Mechanical restraint use and fall-related injuries among residents of skilled nursing facilities. *Annals of Internal Medicine, 116*, 369-374.

Wallach, R. M. (1994). Subacute's success story. *Provider, 20*(10), 51-59.

Waxman, H. M., Carner, E. A., & Berkenstock, G. (1984). Job turnover and job satisfaction among nursing home aides. *The Gerontologists, 24*(5), 503-509.

Young, L. (1989). Pressure ulcer prevalence and associated characteristics in one long-term care facility. *Decubitus, 2*(2), 52.

Zander, K. (1990). Differentiating managed care and case management. *Definition, 5*, 1.

Appendix A

Crude Turnover Rate depicts volume of turnover:

$$\frac{\text{Number (N) of leavers}}{\dfrac{\text{N at start} + \text{N at end}}{2}} \times 100$$

Survival Rate measures the percentage of newly hired personnel who stay.

$$\frac{\text{N of new employees who stay}}{\text{N of new employees}} \times 100$$

Wastage Rate measures the percentage of newly hired personnel who leave.

$$\frac{\text{N of new employees who left}}{\text{N of new employees}} \times 100$$

SOURCE: Duxbury, M. L., & Armstrong, G. D. (1982). Calculating nurse turnover indices. *Journal of Nursing Administration, 12*, 18-24.

CHAPTER 9

Nurses in Transition: A Response to the Changing Health Care System

Ruth M. Tappen   *Patricia Stahura*
Marian C. Turkel   *Frances Morgan*
Rosemary F. Hall

Health care institutions are undertaking significant efforts to reduce costs in the wake of shrinking reimbursement from the government and from private payers. One response to this changing health care environment has been the restructuring of health care delivery systems and the reassignment of nurses from inpatient settings to community-based practice. This chapter describes a cooperative project funded by the Division of Nursing, the University of Miami School of Nursing and Villa Maria/Bon Secours Nursing Center and Rehabilitation Hospital. This project takes an innovative approach to the restructuring issue. In the first phase of the project, staff nurses from the inpatient units learned how to prepare the patient and family for discharge and re-entry into the community. In the second phase, the same nurses visited patients and their families in the home for three months post discharge to ensure successful re-entry into the community and prevent reinstitutionaliza-tion. This chapter provides the perspective of the staff nurse undergoing the

AUTHORS' NOTE: The Nurse-Managed Family Follow-Up in Long-Term Care Project was a study conducted at Villa Maria Nursing and Rehabilitation Center in collaboration with the University of Miami School of Nursing. (Dr. Tappen was a member of the faculty of the University of Miami during this period). This study was supported by a grant funded by the Division of Nursing, Bureau of Health Professions, Department of Health and Human Resources. Correspondence concerning this article should be addressed to Dr. Ruth Tappen at Florida Atlantic University, College of Nursing, 777 Glades Road, Boca Raton, Florida 33431.

transition from the stability of the inpatient setting to the less controlled community environment. The findings from this research serve as a practical example for nursing administrators as they lead and support their nursing staff through transitions in health care delivery.

A funded project designed to support the implementation of an innovative model of nursing practice provided us with the opportunity to observe staff nurses' responses to accomplishing such a transition from inpatient care to community-based care and to analyze the factors that impeded or facilitated the transition. This chapter will critically analyze the issues that arose and discuss strategies to facilitate this type of transition.

The intent of the project was to institute nursing care management and provide follow-up care to patients discharged from the facility by the same nurses who had cared for them as inpatients. The project's unique features were its position in long-term care and the dual role the nurses were expected to assume, providing both inpatient and community-based care.

THE NURSE-MANAGED FAMILY FOLLOW-UP PROJECT

The Project

The Nurse-Managed Family Follow-Up in Long-Term Care Project (NMFF) tested an innovative approach to restructuring nursing practice through a collaborative effort of the University of Miami School of Nursing and Villa Maria Nursing and Rehabilitation Center funded by the Division of Nursing, Department of Health and Human Services. Villa Maria is a 272 bed long-term care facility with 60 CARF-accredited rehabilitation beds and 47 subacute bed. The remainder are long-term care beds. The NMFF Project used staff nurses from the inpatient units of Villa Maria to provide nursing care management to rehabilitation and extended care patients at the facility. The nurses were assigned to patients at the time of admission to the rehabilitation center and assumed responsibility for the management of their care during the patients' stay and for three months postdischarge at home. Faculty from the University of Miami provided direction to the project, education of the nurses, and evaluation of the outcomes of the project.

To create a seamless continuum of care across settings, the same nurse who had provided inpatient care was responsible for assisting the patient and family in making the transition from the nursing center to home. At discharge, the nurse care manager made arrangements to visit the patient within a week after discharge. Follow-up visits continued for the first, second, and third months after the patient went home.

Implementation Plan

Because of the need to spell out project purposes and objectives to obtain funding, we began the project with a clear idea of our goals and the sequence of events that had to occur to achieve those goals. Our implementation plan included the following phases:

1. *Awareness.* All interested parties had to be informed of the project, its purposes and its potential effect on them. This included the patients, families, physicians, home health care agencies, facility social workers, physical therapists, occupational therapists, and the community as a whole.

2. *Organization.* After determining what specific activities would be necessary for implementation of the project, we set target dates for their accomplishment, assigned responsibility for the various tasks, and allocated the resources necessary for their completion (Tappen, 1995).

3. *Education.* Because the staff nurses were primarily diploma and associate degree graduates with many years of inpatient experience but little or no community-based experience, we designed a two-phase classroom and field-based educational program for them to which we later added a third phase of continuing education. Content of the classroom portion included the role of the nursing care manager, family dynamics, cultural diversity, effective communication strategies, community resources (the type available and how to access them) and safety (both home safety for the patient and safety concerns of nurses working in the community).

4. *Operationalization.* Once the nurses were prepared and organizational supports were in place, the inpatient care management and follow-up home care visits by the nurses began.

5. *Formative Evaluation and Modification.* Regular meetings were held with our community advisory board, project consultants, facility administrators, nurse managers, and the staff nurses to monitor progress and modify the plan as needed. Interviews with individual staff nurses at six and eighteen months after initial operationalization were also conducted and proved to be particularly valuable in determining the type of modifications that were necessary.

6. *Summative Evaluation.* End-of-project evaluation included analysis of patient outcome data, organizational impact, economic impact, and staff outcomes. This chapter focuses on the staff outcomes—more specifically, on how successful the nurses were in making the transition to a dual role and what helped and hindered them in making this transition.

In the remainder of this chapter, we will discuss the degree to which the nurses successfully made the transition to a dual role, the issues that were raised as we operationalized this transition, the factors that facilitated the transition and the obstacles to full implementation of the dual role.

THE TRANSITION TO A DUAL ROLE

Prior Experience

Only one of the seven full-time registered nurses involved in the project had any prior home health or public health experience, and that experience had been about 10 years ago in a Western Caribbean country. All the nurses had been inpatient staff nurses for 5 years or more, some for as long as 25 years.

The nurses already had some of the skills that they would need to provide follow-up care postdischarge: familiarity with assistive devices and techniques to promote mobility and self-care, experience teaching patients about the administration of their medications, and dietary modifications, and so forth. The nurses were not accustomed, however, to having to make appointments to see their patients, to working alone in someone else's home, to providing information about community resources, to helping their patients gain access to these resources, to making home environment assessments, or to managing family conflicts. We were asking these institution-based nurses to function in a less structured, more ambiguous setting where the patient might refuse them entry and where guidance from colleagues could be obtained only by telephone or by personal contact later in the day, a sharp contrast to their accustomed routine.

Initial Concerns

A series of meetings was held with the full-time staff nurses to explain the project, its purposes, and their role in it. Although the details of the activities necessary for operationalizing the model had not been worked out yet, we did share a description of the sequence of events that would take place and our vision of the project's potential impact with the nurses.

Because the institution was committed to the project, the staff nurses' involvement was an expectation, not an optional activity. Although they had been hired originally to provide inpatient care, these nurses were suddenly being asked to add community-based care to their practices. They saw this as an addition to their current responsibilities. They expressed concern about an increased workload that stimulated discussion of how well they managed their time and how they could incorporate the follow-up care into their work week.

After these initial meetings with the nurses, we began to hear expressions of both reluctance and insecurity from them. Many were afraid to go out into the community. They were not sure that they wanted to be involved in the project, did not know what they would do in the patient's home or if the patient would want them there, and were not even sure that what we expected them to do was really part of nursing practice.

At first, the nurses found it difficult to approach patients to arrange for follow-up care at home. If a patient elected not to accept the care, they took it personally, hesitating to go back and try again with another patient. As they became more confident, the occasional rejection no longer kept them from approaching other patients. The nurses also learned how to market themselves more effectively by observing the approach used by project staff and by practicing with our guidance.

Another issue the nurses struggled with was some discomfort about going into people's homes. They were concerned that the patients would perceive them as intruders. One said, "sometimes their house is a real mess and it's cluttered and they don't want us to see them in that type of environment." Another added, "They are also tired, they're older, maybe they don't want to have to get the house ready for us to come out and do their visit."

Most of the nurses also had some difficulty adjusting to the idea of going into a patient's home without a detailed procedure for responding to any unexpected problem that might arise. In the home, there was no one present for the nurses to turn to for advice. This apprehension about being on their own is expressed in one of the nurse's comments as she reflected on her initial response to making home visits: "There were no peers to serve as a role model. I was afraid. It loomed over me. I was afraid of making a mistake. There was no one to say, 'I've done this before, do it this way and it will be OK.' "

The nurses were also concerned about their personal safety in unknown and potentially dangerous neighborhoods. Although safety had been discussed in the preparatory classroom sessions, the implications did not sink in until they were ready to go out on their own. To reduce their fear and provide some real assistance in this regard, the safety precautions were reviewed in more detail with them and a cellular telephone was supplied by the institution so that they could call for assistance if necessary.

In the early stages of the transition, the nurses were not certain of their roles as caregivers rather than guests, of the value of making home visits, or of what they had to offer their patients once they left the institution. These insecurities and uncertainties about their role diminished and finally disappeared as they became involved in the care of their patients.

An initial period of dissatisfaction and uneasiness followed by renewed satisfaction has been noted during the implementation of other innovative models of nursing care as well (Kovner, Hendrickson, Knickman, & Finkler, 1994). This may be due to the amount of change and growth demanded of the staff nurses during such a transition. In the NMFF Project, reinforcement of the value of the home visits and of the nurses' competence in conducting them coupled with the clear expectation that they would continue to function in this dual role helped them through this first stage.

Gaining Work Excitement and Satisfaction

Once past the initial insecurity and related concerns, the nurses began to experience what Baldwin and Price (1994) called "work excitement," defined as "enthusiasm and commitment for work as evidenced by creativity, receptivity to learning and ability to see opportunities in everyday situations" (p. 37). The personal and professional rewards and satisfactions they experienced from caring for their patients across the two settings provided them with this work excitement. We believe that it was this feeling that finally transformed them from reluctant participants to enthusiastic supporters of nurse-managed family follow-up care.

The trust relationship that developed between nurse and patient under this new model of nursing care was a key factor in the development of this work satisfaction. The patients knew the nurses from the inpatient setting and felt comfortable sharing details of their personal lives with their nurse care manager. One patient told his nurse, "I'm glad it's you. I don't like strangers in my home. Since it's you, it's OK." The importance of this relationship between patient and nurse was emphasized by all of the staff nurses. It has also been noted in other community-oriented nursing care management projects (Newman, Lamb, & Michaels, 1995).

By following their patients into the community, the nurses were also able to provide an unusual degree of continuity of care. This apparently generated a great deal of comfort for the patients. For example, one patient had fired both the home health nurse and the aide assigned by an outside agency but allowed the nurse care manager to continue visiting. The nurse attributed this to the patient not wanting an unfamiliar person in charge of her care who might try to change her routines: "Since the patients know us, they develop a sense of trust in us. They become used to how you do things, and they don't like a big change in the way things are done. Patients have actually called me their 'security blanket.' Because it is the same nurse from the hospital where the teaching began to following them up at home, the patients don't have to adjust to change," she explained.

The nurses also believed that the patients preferred consistency and did not like having a different nurse on each visit. For example, one nurse said that patients feel that they have accomplished something when they have the same nurse and can do their exercises the way that nurse taught them.

In addition, the nurses felt that establishing a relationship with the patient in the inpatient setting facilitated learning and compliance once the patient was home. It also reduced confusion. When instructions were given by different nurses, the patient often became confused or recalled only the *differences* between the two sets of instructions. With the same nurse, the patient's level of understanding increased at a more rapid rate. Another factor contributing to the creation of work excitement and satisfaction was the opportunity to see that their individual nursing actions made a difference in their patients' lives. One nurse recounted how she prevented a patient from taking an overdose of medication that could have been lethal. Others shared less dramatic but nevertheless satisfying examples of how they had made a difference in their patients' lives. It was apparent that they were making the most of opportunities to intervene effectively with their patients and that they had successfully incorporated home follow-up care into their role of practicing nurse.

IMPEDIMENTS TO SUCCESSFUL TRANSITION

A considerable amount of institutional change was required to accommodate this new dual role for staff nurses. It is evident, both from our observations and from interviews of the nurses involved, that this accommodation is a critical factor in the success of this kind of transition.

The rapid shifts in priorities and financial imperatives of the health care system during project implementation created turbulence for the facility itself. Subsequent to initiation of the project, its corporate owner placed the facility on the market, an event that could not have been foreseen when the project was first proposed. Resources became limited and managers' attention and energies were diverted by the uncertainty regarding the fate of the institution.

Inconsistent Support and Direction

As a result of this organizational turbulence, the amount of support and direction given to the nurses tended to shift with the degree to which managers felt able to direct their energies and resources to the project. For example, the nurses on a particular unit would be told that they were expected to assume the dual role but would not be given sufficient time or flexibility to leave the unit or were limited to certain days of the week convenient to their supervisors but not necessarily to their patients. Pulled in several directions at one time, the nurses became exasperated with this inconsistency.

The transition to a dual role had clear support at the top (administration) and at the bottom (staff nurses) but not in the middle (supervisors) because the middle managers did not have the resources needed for full implementation. Without strong leadership from the top and fully committed managers in the middle, restructuring projects typically flounder and can even fail despite their worthiness in other respects (Hall, Rosenthal, & Wade, 1993). From our interviews with the nurses, it is evident that consistent, firm support and direction would have greatly facilitated their transition and that the inconsistency impeded it. Such inconsistency can occur for any number of reasons other than the institutional turbulence that occurred with this project, including disagreement between various levels of management.

Staffing and Scheduling Demands

Unlike staff nurses in acute care settings who are virtually tied to their assigned units during their shifts, community-based nurses who make home visits need flexible schedules, especially when their patients are not home bound. Scheduling a single staff member for both types of work requires considerable flexibility, ingenuity, and ability to reconcile the care needs of both patient populations. Ultimately, the solution for the NMFF project lay in using a variation of job sharing: Nurse A would be available to the inpatient unit on whatever shift Nurse B was not, and vice versa. This preserved continuity on the unit while allowing the nurses to leave for the purposes of making home visits or taking days off. A more complex form of job sharing among three or more nurses would have been even more flexible but was beyond the capacities of the system.

Making Appointments

Some aspects of the inpatient and community-based roles blended very well. For example, the nurses have learned a great deal about the challenges their patients face when they go home and now incorporate this into inpatient teaching. Other aspects, however, have remained separate, resisting our best attempts to blend them. For example, the nurses found it very difficult to break away from the unit routine long enough to call patients to set up appointments. The nurses were greatly relieved when we offered secretarial assistance for this time-consuming, routine-interrupting task and have expressed their appreciation for this help. It is not the ideal solution, however, as it deprives the nurse and patient of an additional opportunity to maintain communication and continuity after discharge.

Arranging Transportation

When this project was in its planning stages, we met with the staff nurses who would eventually be assuming the dual role, not only to keep them informed but also to obtain their input into design of the model. The majority were interested in the idea but had many questions about the logistics of it.

To our surprise, one staff nurse pointed out that many of the staff do not drive to work. In response, we obtained funding for a rental car to be used by the nurses. This did not solve the problem, however, because many of the nurses did not have a driver's license. This relatively minor problem engendered furious discussion and debate. Should driving skills be required of these nurses? Was it safe to drive alone in some of these neighborhoods? We finally concluded that because driving skills had not been a condition of employment when the nurses were hired, it should not be a requirement now as it did not affect their ability to provide good nursing care, only where they could provide it. Instead, a contract with a local taxi company that would bill monthly was arranged and all the nurses were able to use this mode of transportation.

Although this was a minor problem, it could have endangered the entire project if it had not been solved. Finding a fair but economical solution was critical to maintaining credibility with the staff and to continued forward movement in implementation.

Potential Obstacles

Several anticipated obstacles did not arise, partly because we took steps to prevent them. In particular, we expected some opposition from community-based service organizations and physicians who might assume that the NMFF project was competing with them or would interfere with their function. We found instead that most welcomed the additional guidance afforded the patients and were cooperative once the purpose of the follow-up care was explained. A massive information campaign including numerous meetings and press releases apparently forestalled any potential opposition from these sources.

We also thought that some nurses might find it impossible to make the transition or would find it so unrewarding that they would request removal from the project or resign their positions. In fact, there were no resignations from the nurses who were involved in the project. Although many resisted at first, after they began functioning independently none requested removal or were administratively removed from the project. We believe that the one-to-one clinical mentoring and work excitement that developed were major factors in their commitment to the dual role.

FACILITATING THE TRANSITION

Several strategies facilitated the transition to the dual inpatient-community-based nursing role. Among those already mentioned were having a clear direction and vision of the potential importance of the transition and the willingness to make modifications in the implementation plan as the need arises. The addition of more consistent support and direction from all administrative levels would have greatly facilitated the transition.

The situation in which the institution finds itself is also a critical element in the success of these transitions. Changes within changes can and do occur when transitions are underway. These can present a bewildering set of conflicting expectations to the staff if managers are not clear themselves about their objectives.

Many of the insights reported here came from our interviews with the individual staff nurses who made this transition. A number of problems in need of resolution that we would not otherwise have been aware of were revealed in these interviews. It is of particular interest that these problems had not been brought up in the more public arena of group meetings despite their importance to the nurses. We found the information gained through the interviews to be very valuable and worth the effort for a project of this magnitude.

Our experience with these interviews exemplifies the importance of doing formative as well as summative evaluation. Formative evaluation, that is, evaluation conducted *during* implementation (Morris & Fitz-Gibbon, 1978), provides information at a time when modifications can still be made. Summative evaluation, on the other hand, tells us how well we did and what could have been done more effectively at the end of the project. Our experience also enforces the importance of a *comprehensive* formative evaluation system that includes several different approaches to collecting evaluative feedback and focuses on multiple aspects of the process: the organizational, economic, patient, and individual staff member perspectives. Without it, it would have been difficult, if not impossible, to determine the extent to which implementation was succeeding or failing and why (Hall, Rosenthal, & Wade, 1993).

The educational program designed for this project has been only briefly mentioned but was another key facilitating factor. The three-day intensive classroom portion was considered *necessary* by the nurses but definitely not *sufficient* to prepare them for a major transition.

The classroom portion was followed by individual field experience in the facility and in the home guided by a project staff member who was a clinical specialist in community health. Each staff nurse received individual guidance and coaching on the entire process from initial assessment of the patient and family in the facility through the entire series of home visits. The project staff member acted as a successful role model for nursing care management, provided additional instruction as needed, and reviewed the entire process, including charting, after each visit. The coaching continued until the nurse was ready to function independently. This one-to-one clinical mentoring was the factor most often identified by the nurses themselves as critical to their achieving a successful transition.

Once the nurses began working with patients, the importance of the class-room information became evident to them. In fact, once they became involved in their new roles, the nurses began to ask for more information. This led us to conclude that a third phase of education was also needed.

The third phase of preparation for transition to a new role could be called the continuing education phase. This continuing education should provide more detailed information than was originally provided and opportunities for case discussion and problem solving. For example, the nurses found the infor-mation about community resources overwhelming during the classroom ses-sions. But after they had worked with several patients, they recognized the need for even more information than had been offered during the classroom ses-sions. The relevance of this information had become very clear to them. This also occurred with the personal safety information as well as other topics. Our tentative conclusion is that the initial classroom sessions should include only the essentials needed to assume the new role and that the details should be added after some field experience has been gained.

Finally, the work itself became an important facilitating factor. As the nurses began to do more visits, they gained confidence in their skill and began to recognize the personal and professional satisfaction of being more involved in their patients' lives. Describing how gratifying the dual role was to her, one nurse told us "I have had patients meet me at the bank and say, 'Oh, you were the nurse that helped me.' It gives me such pleasure and I do feel gratified."

DISCUSSION

At the outset, the nurses neither sought nor enthusiastically welcomed the transition thrust on them by the NMFF project. They had been comfortable in their old roles and most wanted to remain in them. They were not prepared either by education or by personal style to adapt to a major change in their role.

In one sense, we asked these experienced nurses to become novices again, to return to finding themselves in clinical situations for which they have had no experience (Benner, 1984). Their early desire for specific procedures and protocols, that is, rules, to guide their practice is an example of this novice behavior. But they moved rapidly through the stages to become proficient if not expert at providing nursing care management and home follow-up care and to incorporate this successfully into a dual inpatient/community-based practice role.

All the strategies discussed in this chapter are useful in helping nurses make such a transition. Of these, firm administrative direction, a three-phase educational program, and the excitement and satisfaction engendered by the work itself seem to be the key factors in achieving a successful transition.

REFERENCES

Baldwin, D. R., & Price, S. A. (1994). Work excitement: The energizer for home health care nursing. *Journal of Nursing Administration, 24* (9), 37-42.

Benner, P. (1984). *From novice to expert: Excellence and power in clinical nursing practice.* Menlo Park, CA: Addison-Wesley.

Hall, G., Rosenthal, J., & Wade, J. (1993). How to make reengineering really work. *Harvard Business Review, 71*(6), 119-131.

Kovner, C., Hendrickson, G., Knickman, J. R., & Finkler, S. A. (1994). Nursing care delivery models and nurse satisfaction. *Nursing Administration Quarterly, 19*(1), 74-85.

Morris, L. L., & Fitz-Gibbon, C. T. (1978). *Educator's handbook.* Beverly Hills: Sage.

Newman, M. A., Lamb, G. S., Michaels, C. (1995). Nurse case management: The coming together of theory and practice. In M. A. Newman (Ed), *A developing discipline: Selected works of Margaret Newman.* New York: National League for Nursing Press.

O'Donnell, K. P., & Sampson, E. M. (1994). Home health care: The pivotal link in the creation of a new health care delivery system. *Journal of Health Care Finance, 21*(2), 74-86.

Peoples, L. T., & Sanders, N. F. (1994). Health care system redesign: A strategic management framework. *Hospital Material Management Quarterly, 16*(2), 1-13.

Tappen, R. M. (1995). *Nursing leadership and management: Concepts and practice* (3rd ed.). Philadelphia: FA Davis.

CHAPTER 10

Advanced Practice Nurses: Key to Successful Hospital Transformation in a Managed-Care Environment

Janet K. Harrison

As hospitals transition from being the hub of the health care system to being service arms of care-managed integrated delivery systems, so too must nurses adapt to the changing health care environment. Advanced practice nurses are contributing in important ways to decreasing acute-care use rates, shortening the length of hospital stays, and improving health outcomes. Although there are exemplary studies demonstrating the effects of nurse interventions on client outcomes and cost of care, lack of scientific rigor characterizes much of this body of literature. The scientific community is challenged to move with haste in demonstrating the added value of the therapeutic actions of clinical nurse specialists and nurse practitioners in a capitated environment.

Advanced practice nurses (APNs) are a critical link in providing cost-effective quality care in the restructured health care delivery system. In heavily managed care environments where integrated delivery systems manage the provision of comprehensive health services for thousands of covered lives, keeping people healthy is the focus. Then when treatment is necessary, the objective is to provide it in the least costly environment where the greatest value can be obtained (Sovie, 1995). Consequently, the focal point of care delivery is rapidly shifting from hospitals to community-based settings.

128

Taking health care to populations in the communities where they live, work, and go to school requires increased numbers of advanced practice nurses to provide primary care and to coordinate care across the health-illness continuum (DeBack & Cohen, 1996). These nurses are a critical link in helping clients adopt healthy lifestyles and use services appropriately along the continuum of care. But nurses must better communicate to others their clinical and economic contributions through outcomes research and cost-benefit analyses. Growing evidence indicates that advanced practice nurses provide care at lower cost than physicians and of equal or superior quality (Office of Technology Assessment, 1986; Safriet, 1992), and that many Americans are willing to receive everyday health care services from nurses (American Nurses Association, 1993). There is also growing evidence that professional nurse case management decreases acute-care admissions, shortens length of hospital stays, lowers health care costs, lessens client-perceived symptom distress and severity of illness, and results in more satisfied clients (Ethridge, 1991; Ethridge & Lamb, 1989; Lamb & Stempel, 1994; Papenhausen, 1996; Sherman & Johnson, 1994).

The purpose of this chapter is to describe the contributions of advanced practice nurses, specifically clinical nurse specialists and nurse practitioners to the successful transformation of the acute-care hospital from revenue-generating center to cost center. Because the first wave of marketplace reform has profoundly influenced the hospital—the workplace of approximately two-thirds of practicing nurses (Donley, 1995)—it was selected as the focal point for this discussion. Three major indicators of successful hospital transformation that advanced practice nurses influence are addressed: acute-care use rates, the length of hospital stays, and health outcomes. Following a brief discussion of the changing practice environment, these influences are described.

THE CHANGING PRACTICE ENVIRONMENT

Capitated managed care in which integrated delivery systems manage the provision of comprehensive health services for thousands of covered lives is becoming prevalent. In metropolitan areas such as Albuquerque, Minneapolis/ St. Paul, Portland, Sacramento, Salt Lake City, and San Diego, a few large integrated systems control more than 50% of the health care market (Lamm, 1994-1995). An integrated system combines physicians, hospitals, and a health plan into one entity that assumes clinical and fiscal responsibility and accountability for providing the full spectrum of services for the enrolled population (Coddington, Moore, & Fischer, 1995; Shortell, 1993). Services are taken to the people through primary care practices distributed geographically throughout the system's service area. The number and mix of specialists and hospital capacity are balanced with the projected number and nature of the health needs of the covered lives. For example, some integrated delivery systems are now operating at 1.5 beds per 1000 members in comparison with the U.S. average of 3.8 per 1000 (Lamm, 1994-1995).

Development of integrated delivery systems closely follows health maintenance organization (HMO) penetration in a given area. The typical payment method used by HMOs is capitation, in which the provider organization receives a negotiated per member per month payment, regardless of whether or not services are accessed and regardless of the type and cost of services received (Alt, 1994). Negotiated portions of the capitated dollar then flow to medical groups and hospitals and are further subdivided for primary and specialty physician services and for inpatient and outpatient hospital services. Withholds from compensation place primary care providers at risk for specialist and hospital referral costs that exceed the referral pools. Once capitation dominates as a payment scheme, hospital use rates and costs drop for all patients as a consequence of health promotion, utilization management, appropriateness standards, and lower-cost modalities (Alt, 1994; O'Donovan, 1994). Because managed care systems aim to meet the needs of subscribers at the lowest possible cost to providers (Porter-O'Grady, 1996), excessive use of hospital services is viewed as a system failure. Hospital survival in a managed care environment requires a steadfast focus on cost reduction, process improvement and value creation (Goldsmith, 1994).

Advanced practice nurses are helping to create a new, cost-effective and high-quality health care system in which health is at the center. Nursing has long championed health promotion, health protection, and disease prevention services as essential to achieving health and wellness and preventing the need for high-intensity medical intervention. Nurses now have the opportunity to demonstrate that health promotion and disease prevention services can prevent the premature onset of disease and disability and help people achieve healthier, more productive lives, which are goals of *Healthy People 2000* (USDHHS, 1991). But nurses need to demonstrate that health promotion and disease prevention services also reduce health care costs. Beginning evidence suggests that advanced practice nurse (APN) interventions are favorably influencing acute-care use rates, length of hospital stays, and health outcomes.

APN INFLUENCES ON ACUTE-CARE USE RATES

The risks assumed under capitation create strong incentives for integrated delivery systems to proactively identify their at-risk or vulnerable populations and reach out to them with programs and services that address their unique needs. In *At Risk in America*, Aday (1993) defined vulnerable populations as those for whom the risk of poor physical, psychological, or social health has or is quite likely to become reality. Those identified as vulnerable include high-risk mothers and infants, the chronically ill and disabled, persons with AIDS, the mentally ill and disabled, and abusing families. Social status (prestige and power), social capital (social support), and human capital (productive potential) place people at greater or lesser risk of poor physical, psychological, or social health (Aday, 1993).

APNs can assist integrated delivery systems in determining the critical screening triggers for identifying health plan subscribers who are vulnerable and at risk of needing high-acuity services. For example, nurse practitioners and certified nurse midwives who care for high-risk mothers and infants know that being a pregnant adolescent minority (social status limitation), an unmarried female head of family (social capital limitation), and poor with less than a high school education (human capital limitation) are predictors of inadequate prenatal care, low birthweight, and infant mortality (Aday, 1993). Through their focus on the biopsychosocial needs, rather than just on physical signs and symptoms, APNs contribute to health-promoting and prevention-oriented care for vulnerable populations such as high-risk mothers and infants. Their community-based primary health services lessen the need for more costly, invasive services.

Coordinating prevention-oriented care for persons in the community is perhaps the greatest contribution that APNs can make to decreasing acute-care use rates. For example, in populations at risk for AIDS, a nurse case manager might coordinate services such as community-based and school-based health education and risk reduction projects, sexual and drug history-taking, substance abuse prevention, safe-sex education, and individual testing and counseling (Aday, 1993). Provision of these services is likely to involve nurses in public health systems, primary care practices, schools, and community-based social agencies. In coordinating the mutually interdependent relationships among the various care providers and practice settings, and over time, the nurse case manager early identifies potential gaps in prevention-oriented care as well as costly duplication of services and takes corrective action.

Each health system needs to make its own determination about who among its covered lives is most vulnerable and likely to benefit from outreach nursing case management services. One community HMO identified its at-risk senior citizens as those who are cognitively and emotionally challenged, have insufficient family support, and have a high probability for sudden physiologic imbalance (Michaels, 1992). When nurse case managers followed these elderly clients over time, monitoring their health status at regular intervals, teaching them to cope with their health concerns, and coordinating medical and community-based support, acute-care use rates declined.

Studies indicate that nurse practitioners are cost-effective providers of primary care services and that there are unique differences between their practice and that of primary care physicians. For example, a meta-analysis of 38 nurse practitioner studies indicated that, in comparison with physician providers, nurse practitioners provided more health promotion activities and scored higher on both quality of care measures and patients' compliance with health promotion and treatment recommendations. In addition, nurse practitioners spent more time with patients than did physicians and their patients experienced fewer hospitalizations (Brown & Grimes, 1993). These findings must be interpreted with caution because most of the studies were conducted during the 1970s when lack of scientific rigor characterized many of the studies.

Studies also indicate that advanced practice nurse interventions with acute-care, nursing home, and home health patients can assist integrated delivery systems in controlling hospital use rates. Several clinical trials have demonstrated the effects of specific clinical nurse specialist interventions on hospitalization and rehospitalization. Naylor, Brooten, Jones, Lavizzo-Mourey, Mezey, and Pauley (1994) found that elderly cardiac patients receiving comprehensive discharge planning by a gerontological clinical nurse specialist had fewer readmissions in the six-week period following discharge than the control group. Findings from the Robert Wood Johnson Foundation Teaching Nursing Home program revealed that geriatric clinical nurse specialist and nurse practitioner direct care interventions in nursing homes resulted in a 7% decline in hospital admission rates compared with a 5% increase in matched comparison nursing homes (Shaughnessy, Kramer, & Hittle, 1990). McCorkle, Benoliel, Donaldson, Georgiadon, Moinpour, and Godell (1989) found that adult patients with progressive lung disease who received home care from an oncological clinical nurse specialist had fewer hospital admissions for malignancy-related symptoms and complications than patients who either did not receive home care or received it from home health nurses. Positive fiscal outcomes are also a result of nurse interventions that shorten hospital stays.

APN INFLUENCES ON THE LENGTH OF HOSPITAL STAYS

To assist integrated delivery systems in controlling length of hospital stays, clinical nurse specialists must expand and more fully use all components of their role: practice, teaching, consultation, research, and administration (ANA, 1984). Reductions in hospital length of stay as a consequence of clinical nurse specialist interventions were reported by Brooten and Naylor (1995). Interventions of a perinatal clinical nurse specialist resulted in very low-birth weight infants being discharged a mean of 11.2 days earlier than control group infants, with no significant differences in rehospitalization rates (Brooten et al., 1986). Lipman (1986) found that interventions of a clinical nurse specialist resulted in newly diagnosed diabetic children being discharged a mean of 2.2 days earlier than children cared for solely by staff nurses, with no differences in rehospitalization rates. Neidlinger, Scroggins, and Kennedy (1987) found that implementation of a comprehensive discharge planning protocol by a gerontological clinical nurse specialist resulted in a two-day reduction in length of hospital stay for elders 75 years of age and older, in comparison with control group patients who received routine discharge planning by the primary nurse.

Achievement of clinical outcomes within preestablished standards for hospital length of stay has resulted in the proliferation of acute-care case management models. In most of the models presented in the literature, the primary nurse at the bedside assumes responsibility for ensuring that the multidisciplinary plan of care is relevant for the specific patient and carried out in the most timely and cost-effective manner (Cohen & Cesta, 1994). Studies have shown that acute-care case management results in shorter lengths of hospital stay; however, statistically significant differences are reported infrequently. Cohen (1991) found significant differences in length of stay of cesarean-section patients when clinical pathways were used. Sperry and Birdsall (1994) found significant differences in length of stay before and after introduction of a pneumonia clinical path. An analysis of the research on hospital-based nursing case management led McCloskey and colleagues (1994) to conclude that little scientifically rigorous research is available to demonstrate cost and quality effectiveness of case management.

Although monitoring resource use and adherence to the clinical pathway and care map will likely, in the future, become standard practice for all hospitalized patients, case management services are better reserved for select patient groups who are at risk for variances from the standards. Clinical nurse specialists have the requisite knowledge and skills to direct the case management program for these at-risk populations. Advanced academic preparation for nurse case managers is advocated by many authors (Gibson, Martin, Johnson, Blue, & Miller, 1994; Sherman & Johnson, 1994; Trinidad, 1993). Advanced practice nurses can be the process and resource consultants for the direct care providers. In addition, they can troubleshoot recurring variances from established pathways, collaborate with providers across the continuum of care, and investigate cost and quality effectiveness of case management. As clinical nurse specialists expand and more fully use all the roles they have been prepared to assume, they will be perceived as indispensable to the provision of high-quality cost-effective acute care in hospitals.

The professional nurse case management (PNCM) model at Carondelet Hospitals and Medical Centers in Tuscon, Arizona, has been the focus of several studies involving chronically ill, elderly clients. Central to the success of this advanced practice dominated model is formation of a therapeutic nurse-client relationship from which mutually derived client outcomes emerge (Papenhausen, 1996). In a partnership with the high-risk client, the professional nurse case manager moves with the client across the spectrum of health care helping the client to live with one or more chronic diseases (Michaels, 1992). Shorter length of stays have been reported using this continuum of care model that blends elements of acute and community case management. Ethridge (1991) reported that enrollees in a nursing HMO for seniors had shorter length of hospital stays than a comparison group of Medicare patients. Comparing case-managed high-risk patients against lower acuity controls, Ethridge and Lamb (1989) reported a two-day reduction in length of stay as a result of professional nurse case management. Using the PNCM model at a midwestern medical center, average length of stay was decreased by 31% (Rogers, Reardon, & Swindle, 1991). The model has also been used to case manage chronically ill subjects in a northern midwest state. Gibson et al. (1994) reported reduced length of stays following six-months of case management in comparison with the six-month period before implementation of PNCM. Several nurse researchers have proposed that the cost benefits of decreased hospitalizations and lengths of stays are linked to health outcomes (Ethridge, 1991; Ethridge & Lamb, 1989; Michaels, 1992; Papenhausen, 1996).

APN INFLUENCES ON HEALTH OUTCOMES

According to Carlson (1995), measures that truly reflect health, such as function enhancement, social and emotional wellness, vitality, lifestyle, and preventive measures, must replace the old standards that evolved around "dishealth"—morbidity, mortality, and complications. Mortality and morbidity measures provide little understanding of the effects of nursing interventions, according to Brooten and Naylor (1995), who called for investigation of health outcomes that are more sensitive to nursing actions.

Review of the recent literature revealed only a few studies on the influence of advanced practice nurse interventions on nurse-sensitive health outcomes. Papenhausen (1996) measured client outcomes before and after three months of professional nurse case management interventions in a sample of 76 chronically ill high-risk adults. Nurse case management interventions resulted in significant decreases in client-perceived severity of illness, perceived physical disability, and perceived symptom distress. Analysis of qualitative data from a subset of the main sample revealed client statements supporting decreased severity of illness, decreased perception of physical disability, and improved symptom management. Burgess, Lerner, D'Agostino, Vokonas, Hartman, and Gaccione (1987) found that three months postdischarge, myocardial infarction patients who received psychosocial rehabilitation from a clinical nurse specialist were significantly less distressed psychologically and less dependent on family support than control subjects. In assessing the effects of home care provided by oncological nurse specialists, McCorkle, et al. (1989) found statistically significant less system distress and greater independence in those receiving home care than in the control group not receiving home care.

CONCLUSION

The roles of advanced practice nurses are in transition as the nursing profession responds to the growing pressure for more cost-effective and consumer-responsive managed care. Increased numbers of clinical nurse specialists and nurse practitioners are delivering front-line care in community-based settings, which is reducing the need for costly, invasive procedures and hospital days. These nurses are creating partnerships with individuals and communities and empowering them to take more responsibility for their own health. New functions that have evolved for which nurses are uniquely suited include benefits interpreter, case manager, client advocate, resource manager, risk manager, and primary care provider (Barter, Graves, Phoon, & Corder, 1995). Califano (1994) suggested that as much as 80% of the primary care that family physicians normally provide could be safely delivered by nonphysician providers. Perhaps now is the time for advanced practice nurses to seize the opportunity to be the first tier providers of primary care, who refer the more complex cases to primary care physicians, who in turn are the gatekeepers to physician specialists (Califano, 1994).

More research adds to the credibility and perceived value of clinical nurse specialists and nurse practitioners. Some exemplary clinical trials have demonstrated the effects of clinical nurse specialist interventions on hospitalization and rehospitalization rates, length of hospital stays, and selected patient outcomes. Research on the effects of advanced practice nurse interventions on client outcomes such as health-promoting behaviors, self-care status, and well-being is in its infancy.

Methodological shortcomings characterize many of the studies of nurse practitioner effectiveness. Physician care has been the standard to which nurse practitioner care has been compared. Using physician care as the gold standard suggests that support for the substitution of nurse practitioners for physicians in the provision of primary care was the primary aim at the time the research was conducted. What is now needed are clinical trials to investigate the effects of nurse practitioner interventions on health-promoting behaviors, social and emotional wellness, and lifestyle self-management, outcomes that can substantially reduce health care costs as a result of fewer acute-care hospitalizations and shorter hospital stays.

Some nurse leaders argue for blending the roles of clinical nurse specialist and nurse practitioner into one advanced practice role (Mallison, 1993; Porter-O'Grady, 1996; Schroer, 1991). Others are concerned that nursing might be selling itself short by identifying the predominant advanced practice role of the future as a primary care provider rather than as a clinical expert and leader (Beecroft, 1994; Betz, 1994). Until scientifically rigorous research is conducted, it seems unwise to blend the roles into a model that contributes more to the traditional role of medicine rather than to nursing and health care. The scientific community is challenged to move with haste in demonstrating the added value of the therapeutic actions of advanced practice nurses in a capitated environment.

REFERENCES

Aday, L. A. (1993). *At risk in America.* San Francisco: Jossey-Bass.

Alt, S. J. (1994). HMOs demand better hospital deals as markets shift to managed care. *Health Care Strategic Management, 12*(4), 9-10.

American Nurses Association (ANA). (1984). *Issues in professional nursing practice: Specialization in nursing practice.* Kansas City: ANA.

American Nurses Association. (1993, December 9). *News Release.* Washington, DC: ANA.

Barter, M., Graves, J., Phoon, J., & Corder, K. (1995). The changing health care delivery structure: Opportunities for nursing practice and administration. *Nursing Administration Quarterly, 19,* 74-80.

Beecroft, P. C. (1994). CNS: Thriving or heading for extinction? *Clinical Nurse Specialist, 8,* 63.

Betz, C. L. (1994). Is nursing selling itself short? *Journal of Pediatric Nursing, 9,* 139-140.

Brooten, D., Kumar, S., Butts, P., Finkler, S., Bakewell-Sachs, S., Gibbons, A., & Delivoria-Papadopoulos, M. (1986). A randomized clinical trial of early hospital discharge and home follow-up of very low birth weight infants. *New England Journal of Medicine, 315,* 934-939.

Brooten, D., & Naylor, M. D. (1995). Nurses' effect on changing patient outcomes. *Image, 27,* 95-99.

Brown, S. A., & Grimes, D. E. (1993). *Nurse practitioners and certified nurse midwives: A meta-analysis of studies on nurses in primary care roles.* Washington, DC: American Nurses Publishing.

Burgess, A. W., Lerner, D. J., D'Agostino, R. B., Vokonas, P. S., Hartman, C. R., & Gaccione, P. (1987). A randomized control trial of cardiac rehabilitation. *Social Science Medicine, 24,* 359-370.

Califano, J. A. (1994). *Radical surgery: What's next for America's health care.* New York: Random House.

Carlson, L. K. (1995). The next step. *Healthcare Forum Journal, 38*(3), 14-18.

Coddington, D. C., Moore, K. D., Fischer, E. A. (1995). Integrating? Hang in there—The odds are in your favor. *Healthcare Forum Journal, 38*(1), 72-76.

Cohen, E. (1991). Nursing case management: Does it pay? *Journal of Nursing Administration, 21*(4), 20-25.

Cohen, E. L., & Cesta, T. G. (1994). Case management in the acute care setting. *Journal of Case Management, 3*, 110-116, 128.

DeBack, V., & Cohen, E. (1996). The new practice environment. In E. L. Cohen (Ed.), *Nurse case management in the 21st century* (pp. 3-9). St. Louis: Mosby.

Donley, R. (1995). Advanced practice nursing after health care reform. *Nursing Economic$, 13*, 84-88, 98.

Ethridge, P. (1991). A nursing HMO: Carondelet St. Mary's experience. *Nursing Management, 22*(7), 22-27.

Ethridge, P., & Lamb, G. (1989). Professional nursing case management improves quality, access and costs. *Nursing Management, 20*(3), 30-35.

Gibson, S. J., Martin, S. M., Johnson, M. B., Blue, R., & Miller, D. S. (1994). CNS-directed case management: Cost and quality in harmony. *Journal of Nursing Administration, 24*, 45-51.

Goldsmith, J. C. (1994). The illusive logic of integration. *Healthcare Forum Journal, 37*(5), 26-31.

Lamb, G. S., & Stempel, J. E. (1994). Nurse case management from the client's view: Growing as insider-expert. *Nursing Outlook, 41*, 7-13.

Lamm, R. (Winter, 1994-1995). The ghost of health care future. *Inquiry, 31*, 365-367.

Lipman, T. (1986). Length of hospitalization of children with diabetes: Effect of clinical nurse specialist. *The Diabetes Educator, 14*, 41-43.

Mallison, M. (1993). Nurses as house staff. *American Journal of Nursing, 93*, 7.

McCloskey, J. C., Mass, M., Huber, D. G., Kasparek, A., Specht, J., Ramler, C., Watson, C., Blegen, M., Delaney, C., Ellerbe, S., Etscheidt, C., Gongaware, C., Johnson, M., Kelly, K., Mehmert, P., & Clougherty, J. (1994). Nursing management innovations: A need for systematic evaluation. *Nursing Economic$, 12*(1), 35-44.

McCorkle, R., Benoliel, J., Donaldson, G., Georgiadon, F., Moinpour, C., & Godell, B. (1989). A randomized clinical trial of home nursing care for lung cancer patients. *Cancer, 64*, 1375-1382.

Michaels, C. (1992). Carondelet St. Mary's nursing enterprise. *Nursing Clinics of North America, 27*, 77-85.

Naylor, M., Brooten, D., Jones, R., Lavizzo-Mourey, R., Mezey, M., & Pauly, M. (1994). Comprehensive discharge planning for hospitalized elderly: A randomized clinical trial. *Annals of Internal Medicine, 120*, 999-1006.

Neidlinger, L., Scroggins, K., & Kennedy, L. (1987). Cost evaluation of discharge planning for hospitalized elderly. *Nursing Economic$, 5*, 225-230.

O'Donovan, P. (1994). Making the transition to a new environment requires forethought and planning. *Health Care Strategic Management, 12*(8), 15-17.

Office of Technology Assessment. (1986). *Health technology case study 37. Nurse practitioners, physician assistants, and certified nurse-midwives: A policy analysis.* Washington, DC: Congress of the United States.

Papenhausen, J. L. (1996). Discovering and achieving client outcomes. In E. L. Cohen (Ed.), *Nurse case management in the 21st century* (pp. 257-268). St. Louis: Mosby.

Porter-O'Grady, T. (1996). Nurses as advanced practitioners and primary care providers. In E. L. Cohen (Ed.), *Nurse case management in the 21st century* (pp. 10-20). St. Louis: Mosby.

Rogers, M., Riordan, J., & Swindle, D. (1991). Community-based nursing case management pays off. *Nursing Management, 22*(3), 30-34.

Safriet, B. J. (1992). Health care dollars and regulatory sense: The role of advanced practice nursing. *Yale Journal on Regulation, 9*(2), 417-418.

Schroer, K. (1991). Case management: Clinical nurse specialist and nurse practitioner, converging roles. *Clinical Nurse Specialist, 5,* 189-194.

Shaughnessy, P., Kramer, A., & Hittle, D. (1990, March). *The teaching nursing home experiment, its effect and implications.* Study Paper 6. Center for Health Services Research, University of Colorado.

Sherman, J. J., & Johnson, P. K. (1994). CNS as unit-based case manager. *Clinical Nurse Specialist, 8,* 76-80.

Shortell, S. M. (1993). Creating organized delivery systems: The barriers and facilitators. *Hospital and Health Services Administration, 38*(4), 447-466.

Smith, M. C. (1995). The core of advanced practice nursing. *Nursing Science Quarterly, 8,* 2-3.

Sovie, M. D. (1995). Tailoring hospitals for managed care and integrated health systems. *Nursing Economic$, 13,* 72-83.

Sperry, S., & Birdsall, C. (1994). Outcomes of a pneumonia critical path. *Nursing Economic$, 12,* 332-339, 345.

Trinidad, E. A. (1993). Case management: A model of CNS practice. *Clinical Nurse Specialist, 7,* 221-223.

U.S. Department of Health and Human Services (USDHHS). (1991). *Healthy people 2000: National health promotion and disease prevention objectives* (USDHHS Publication No. (PHS) 91-50212). Washington, DC: Government Printing Office.

CHAPTER 11

Clinical Nurse Specialists: The Third Generation

K. Sue Haddock

Clinical nurse specialists (CNSs) have evolved over time from direct caregivers to a combination educator-researcher-consultant. But given the emerging constraints in today's health care, the CNS role must change. Unfortunately, in today's health care environment, CNSs have been marked for extinction because of their high price tag and poorly marketed role. CNSs are valuable resources, however; resources nurse administrators *need* to facilitate quality, cost-effective care.

Nurse practitioners and case managers are two roles receiving widespread acceptance in health care and having potential for transitioning CNSs. Both roles are worthy of consideration as nurse administrators ponder the question of what to do with their CNSs. Regardless of which role is chosen, CNSs will need to be proactive, and nurse administrators will need to assist CNSs make the transition for success under health care reform and managed care.

Managed care discussions in health care have precipitated a flurry of cost-containment and role restructuring in health care systems. As the nation struggles with health care reforms for the provision of accessible and affordable health care, nurse administrators must examine nursing roles for the changing environment (Forbes, 1992). Quality care will require appropriately linking nurses with patient needs, both within and outside acute care settings.

AUTHOR'S NOTE: Special acknowledgment to four nurses who were willing to share their joys and frustrations of being in the CNS role: Hannah L. Holmes, MN, RNC, CS; Katie G. Roach, MS, RN, CS; Nancy L. Smith, MN, RNC, CS; Katherine Kenan, RNC, MSN, CNS.

139

Clinical nurse specialists (CNSs) are one group of nurses with advanced skills who have traditionally delivered care within the hospital and who have a strong history of positively affecting patient care outcomes. Why then, are many hospitals eliminating CNS positions (Lynn-McHale, Fitzpatrick, & Shaffer, 1993)? The answer is complex, but before nurse administrators agree to dispense with these positions, they must examine why the CNS role was created and consider how nurses currently in these roles can best be used in the evolving system of managed care.

FIRST GENERATION CNS

The first generation CNS position was established in 1969 at the University of Virginia Medical Center. The intent behind the development of the CNS role was to provide nursing staff with an expert who had clinical, educational, consulting, and research skills. This specialist would be able to reduce costs and improve patient care (Burge, Crigler, Hurt, Kelly, & Sanborn, 1989). During this time, considerable literature was written on the effectiveness of CNSs, but other literature expressed concerns about the overwhelming responsibilities associated with such an encompassing role (Minarik, 1990). As nurse administrators struggled with the most effective use of CNSs, a variety of responsibilities emerged. The deployment and the job-associated duties for CNSs varied among employing institutions, resulting in considerable confusion about the role (Page & Arena, 1994).

The dialogue about what the CNS actually does in day-to-day practice continued. Holt (1987) noted that CNSs spent a greater percentage of time on consultation versus clinical practice and that as the CNS became more seasoned in the role, more time was spent in scholarly activities. Walker (1986) asked CNSs to estimate time spent in each of the role areas and reported that more than 50% of the time, regardless of experience in the role, was spent on patient care and consultation. A report by Burge and colleagues (1989), on data collected over four years, concurred with Walker's summary of CNS activities, finding that CNSs with more experience in the role spent approximately 30% of their time in consultation compared with 16% consulting time spent by CNSs with less experience. Neophyte CNSs devoted 44% of their time to direct patient care activities, 25% of their time in educational efforts, and the remaining 15% in scholarly and miscellaneous activities.

SECOND GENERATION CNS

In the mid 1980s, the second generation CNS emerged. Changes in health care reimbursement, shifts from quality care to quality/cost-balanced care caused CNSs to expand from the nurse and patient focus to an organization and system focus. This second generation CNS's academic background often included courses on systems theory, administrative decision making, cost accounting and analysis, reimbursement systems, and the art and science of nursing. CNSs began to address factors contributing to patient care outcomes, problems contributing to ineffective nursing practice, and programs that supported a resource-driven model of care (Wolf, 1990).

The second generation CNSs were largely successful because of their system orientation. CNSs identified and corrected systemwide factors contributing to problematic patient outcomes and ineffective or inefficient nursing practice (Wolf, 1990). Furthermore, CNSs developed strategies to modify practice requirements and cost-effective innovations in delivery systems, thus enhancing quality patient care. During this time, CNSs developed the knowledge base and effectively implemented changes in practice that resulted in substantial decreases in length of stay for elderly patients (Kennedy, Niedlinger, & Scroggins, 1987), low birthweight infants (Brooten, Gennara, Knapp, Jovene, Brown, & York, 1991) and cardiac patients (Wolf, 1990). CNSs also established health promotion programs and programs to prevent patient falls and decubitus ulcers.

The role of the CNS seemed firmly established. Graduate programs marketing CNS programs were abundant. Certification examinations were developed to certify CNSs in many clinical specialties. In the work place, however, issues continued to surface that focused on what these expensive professionals really did and were they really worth the dollar expenditures? Again, the central issue appeared to be confusion about the actual role responsibilities. Clearly, members of various health care professions had different expectations. Nurse administrators wanted clinical experts who could provide clinical leadership, orient new staff, conduct research on clinical problems and save the organization money. Staff nurses expected CNSs to be clinical experts who could relieve them of some of their clinical responsibilities. Physicians weren't sure what to expect: Was this another staff nurse with a fancy title or a stand-in head nurse? Fenton (1985) suggested that the CNS job description should be developed for the specific needs of the organization and based on the competencies required to implement the role within the institution. Unfortunately, this actually happened and has resulted in CNS job descriptions differing from setting to setting, again adding to role confusion.

A recent review of current undergraduate leadership and graduate nursing administration textbooks revealed that the role of the CNS is not even addressed (Gillies, 1994; Simms, Price, & Ervin, 1994; Tappen, 1995; Yoder Wise, 1995). Only one textbook, of those reviewed, listed the clinical nurse specialist in the index (Vestal, 1995). None of the books included the CNS as a member of the care team or even as an adjunct to nursing staff. Perhaps this lack of attention in the resources used to educate nurses in leadership roles reflects the existing role confusion and lack of clear vision about how to integrate CNSs into the nursing system.

The pervasive vagueness about the composite role also has contributed to confusion within the CNS group and to perceived devaluation by both nursing and hospital administration. Role responsibilities for research and consultation are not readily appreciated by staff nurses and ambiguous clinical obligations have frustrated both nursing and hospital administration when trying to identify clinical costs per patient. The financial personnel, who tend to look at reports for only the "bottom line," have difficulty justifying the need for someone who does not have a well-defined role with expected outcomes that either increase profitability or decrease cost (Neidlinger, Scroggins, & Kennedy, 1987). The result of devaluation of the CNS role has been a decrease in the number of CNS positions, reclassification of job responsibilities of CNSs, frustration in academic centers about how to prepare CNSs to meet the multiple expectations, and confusion among the existing CNS group about future job security.

THIRD GENERATION CNS

The health care system is undergoing some drastic changes. One element has remained constant, however—the continued emphasis on cost containment. The new approach to cost containment is "managed care." The success of managed care seems to rely on the assumption that health care costs are out of control because no one has managed care in the past! What managed care really seems to mean is that health care will go through *reengineering* and emerge with new management to control all costs associated with patient services. Given this as the reality for health care, there will be winners and losers depending on how well one can control financial outcome (and quality ones, it is hoped). For nursing to survive in the managed care environment, nurses must be able to coordinate multidisciplinary plans for patient care, navigate the financial domains for reimbursements that either provide maximum return or reduce the amount of loss, assess the patient and family socioeconomic situation, and factor that into the overall plan of care and manage the patient's continuum of care. Practice in the hospital-based managed care arena clearly calls for nurses with advanced practice skills and a broad understanding of the health care system to integrate and coordinate the multidisciplinary services required throughout the patient's illness episode (Allred, Arford, Michel, Dring, Carter,

& Veitch, 1995). One cannot help but speculate that nurse administrators have a golden opportunity to reframe the CNS role into the third generation CNS. Two options present themselves for consideration: development of CNSs into nurse practitioners or progression of CNSs to case managers. Both options are presented.

NURSE PRACTITIONER

Reframing the role of the CNS as a nurse practitioner is the first option to be discussed. The nurse practitioner role has long been established in the delivery of primary health services. Nurse practitioners have functioned well in practitioner-run clinics, physician offices, and other ambulatory settings. Recently, there has been interest in expanding the use of nurse practitioners to acute care settings. Academic institutions now offer graduate programs preparing nurses to work as acute care nurse practitioners (ACNP).

Students are prepared for the acute care role through a graduate curriculum with the standard core of research, theory, issues, and statistics courses, then fill the remainder of requirements with advanced physical assessment, pharmacology, advanced pathophysiology, and clinically relevant topics (with practicums). These programs are completed in 39 to 45 hours of graduate education. Although the focus of many of these programs is on the adult, clinical practicums allow some specialization with a particular population such as pediatrics, geriatrics, oncology, and mental health.

For clinical nurse specialists who already have a graduate degree, postmasters certificate programs are being offered in which courses augment previous graduate work and prepare students for the nurse practitioner role. An average of 18 hours of course work is required to prepare these nurses to function in the acute care setting in lieu of the house medical officer or in conjunction with a physician's private practice but focusing on the needs of hospitalized patients. Another site interested in ACNP, because of the economic impact, are long-term care providers who previously have had physician coverage.

Nurse practitioners have prescriptive authority, reimbursement privileges, and a legal scope of practice. Currently, nurse practitioners have some measure of prescribing authority in 43 states. Under Medicaid, 42 states have allowed reimbursement for nurse practitioner services. Medicare reimbursement is permitted in 18 states for certain services and was extended to practitioner services provided by nurses in nursing facilities in 1990 (American College of Physicians, 1994). Clearly, the role of the nurse practitioner is receiving widespread acceptance in primary care and nursing home settings. The role adaptation for the acute care setting is anticipated to receive similar acceptance.

For nurse administrators interested in this option, the CNS needs to be supported in the preparation for the role change. Support can come via tuition reimbursement, release time for course work or flex-time, and the identification of practice sites within the organization. For effectiveness, positions for acute care nurse practitioners need to be developed and embedded in the structure. Nurse administrators also need to clearly articulate this role to organizational members to avoid the role confusion that previously plagued CNSs. Successful implementation of this role will depend heavily on acceptance by the medical staff. In some states, nurse practitioners must have a physician supervisor, so it is essential that physicians are approached about the proposed changes early. Using physician preceptors during the educational process will help with acceptance of the role. Information sessions must be conducted for both medical staff and other members of the health care system (pharmacists, social workers, finance personnel, nurses, etc.) to prepare them for the changes. Physician preceptors can be involved in case studies illustrating how the nurse practitioner can augment and enhance patient care. These strategies are especially useful while the role is being developed within the organization and while the CNS is still involved in the academic preparation. The nurse administrator will want to carefully consider placement options for the new nurse practitioners and place them where they will be able to use their new skills and where they will be able to develop a close relationship with other members of the health care team. Such areas include critical care units, the emergency room, and ambulatory care clinics for both pediatric and adult populations.

The nurse practitioner option is viable as a survival technique for CNSs if nurse administrators carefully orchestrate the changing role with the support and input from faculty in academic institutions, CNSs, physicians, and other administrators in the organization. CNSs will need to adapt to a changed role with new functions and duties. If all systems are attended to properly, however, CNSs should experience a successful role transition.

CASE MANAGER

Case management was a nursing role early in the development of the profession. Recently, the role has been reengineered to complement the current health care system. Case management is intended to result in collaborative multidisciplinary nurse-coordinated care that is cost-effective and accountable. Case management as a delivery model in the 1990s answers the demand for provision of high-quality care in a cost-effective manner (Lynn-McHale et al., 1993). The case manager (CM) integrates clinical and management skills with professional and financial accountability to ensure that needed health care resources are accessible and available at a reasonable cost.

Nurses prepared as case managers focus on collaboration and consultation among disciplines. Because of the emphasis on collaboration and consultation skills, nurses with master's level clinical expertise and knowledge of evaluation need to be selected as case managers. Master's level nurses are more likely to use problem-solving processes to identify and resolve problems across patient groups, collaborate among all components of the hospital system and evaluate the clinical and financial impact of the case management strategies (Brockopp, Porter, Kinnaird, & Silberman, 1992). Costs can be reduced without increasing morbidity and mortality by using the CM to affect the nursing management of patient populations (Soehren & Schumann, 1994; Strong, 1992). The CM is the ideal person to coordinate care across settings such as the hospital system, outpatient clinics or the home. As a case manager, the CNS can minimize fragmentation by mobilizing multidisciplinary resources and making system-level changes to enhance care and outcomes (Strong, 1992).

To nurture case managers, nurse administrators must be willing to devote significant energies and resources into a case management program. Case management requires multidisciplinary collaboration with physicians playing key roles. As with developing a nurse practitioner role, physicians must be brought into the plans for change at a very early stage. Other professionals needed early in the program planning include social workers and utilization review personnel. Often this can result in "turf" battles and must be handled diplomatically. In addition, the CNSs becoming case managers must take responsibility for developing the skills necessary for the role and must be willing to identify indicators of their effect on patient outcomes. During this transition time, the nurse administrator must keep the concept of organizational viability clearly in the open and continue to demonstrate commitment to that view, being careful to never allow the suspicion to surface that CNSs are just being given new titles to survive reengineering.

Unlike the nurse practitioner, case managers do not have a specially designed graduate program or postmaster's certificate. Courses may be offered at the local university, however, that address many of the role elements and responsibilities. Nurse administrators will want to encourage their CNSs to take advantage of such courses. If courses are not available, numerous conferences address role preparation for case management. Another option the nurse administrator could pursue is providing professional development workshops for CNSs. These workshops can be led by case managers from other organizations. Because of the diversity in case management programs, the nurse administrator will want to carefully select a model to replicate. Consultation with the CNSs and a variety of stakeholders will enhance the model choice and implementation.

Once a case management model is chosen, a project director must be identified. The chosen case management model will need to be clearly described and articulated to the organization. Although CNSs will need development and support during this stressful period of change, the results for the organization in fiscal and patient outcomes will be worth the struggle.

EXISTING EXAMPLES

Currently, this author is consulting with two organizations who are attempting to redefine the roles of their CNSs and managing within a third organization that is reexamining the need for the CNS. The first organization has systematically moved in the direction of case management. In developing their program, this organization identified a project manager who has worked with the CNS group to clearly define the role of the case manager within the organization's system. Several CNSs have elected to return to school for courses on the acute care practitioner track. Others have chosen to attend workshops and seminars on the role and functions of case managers.

The largest obstacle the CNSs have encountered comes from within themselves as each tries to sort out the differences between what they *had* been doing as CNSs and what they are now *expected* to be doing as case managers. The role of nurse practitioner has not been promoted within this acute care setting as an option for the CNSs. Nurse practitioners are being hired for the emergency department and by several physician practice groups, however. The nurse administrator in this setting is a strong proponent for CNSs moving into the case manager role and has had this role presented to and accepted by both hospital administration and physicians. Much work by the nurse administrator led to this acceptance. Having a clearly defined and communicated role for the transitioning CNSs was key to this success. Work is now in progress to evaluate the patient and organizational outcomes of this change. Information from patient satisfaction surveys, follow-up telephone calls to discharged patients, length of stay data, and hospital charges data will be used for evaluation purposes.

A second hospital also elected to transition CNSs into case managers. Unfortunately, this hospital has not made the same effort to define the role and make it part of the accepted delivery system. There has been no project director, and there has been little support of CNSs returning to school for either case management skills or nurse practitioner skills. CNSs transitioning to case management are struggling with some of the same problems of role confusion as well as poor understanding of the role by others in the organization. The new case managers are frustrated with trying to identify and function in a new role while still being responsible for many of the tasks from the CNS role. Administrative support is obviously needed as well as a specific method for demonstrating the case managers' effectiveness. CNSs in the second organization are very concerned about their viability within a system that does not understand either the CNS or the case manager role.

In the third organization, the nurse executive is attempting to create a role for nurses with advanced practice skills to function as either a case manager or as a nurse practitioner. Attracting nurses with advanced degrees has been problematic because of the perceived low pay scales in this state's mental health acute care (medical/surgical) hospital. At this point, the nurse executive is willing to support either role and will make a choice when a suitable candidate is identified. Administration and physicians have had both roles described to them and the need for nurses working in these advanced roles. Both groups are willing to accept either role and would actually support both roles if the budget would allow! Communication about the new role has been instrumental in this acceptance as well as arranging for a geriatric nurse practitioner (GNP) faculty member to precept ACNP students within the facility. The GNP worked with physician staff to identify learning opportunities for students and encouraged medical staff to become involved with the students' experiences.

CONCLUSIONS

Research on the effectiveness of CNSs in the care of high risk patient populations (Brooten et al., 1991; Kennedy et al., 1987) has demonstrated that clinical nurse specialists are a precious and valuable resource in health care. In times of extreme pressures to cut costs, it is often tempting to eliminate expensive members of an organization, that is, the CNS. The research on outcomes associated with nurses in advanced practice roles provides nurse administrators proactive information to defend and protect these roles. Clearly, some of the best "buys" in health care today are in the form of CNSs. To proactively respond to the emerging demands in health care, however, the nurse administrator may need to assist CNSs moving into either a nurse practitioner or case manager role. Within these roles, CNSs will have even more of the skills needed to meet the demands of managed care and health care reform. Although preservation of CNSs will depend largely on the commitment of nurse administrators to advanced practice roles in the acute care setting, the CNSs also must be willing to develop skills that demonstrate their innovation, centrality, and effectiveness.

Nurse administrators must take a long, hard look at how CNSs currently function within the organization and ask whether the CNS role is really giving the organization what is needed. If the answer is no, then both the CNSs and the nurse administrator must be prepared to make changes. Two options were presented that give nurse administrators direction in making needed changes to enhance cost-effective, quality patient care. In either role, CNSs can provide clinical care as needed for selected patients, model expert care to develop staff nurses, act as a consultant to nurse managers for identification and implementation of needed system changes, and conduct research to evaluate the practitioner or case management models. All components of the CNS role can easily be incorporated into the third generation role but in a way that clarifies the role to the public, to other nurses, to physicians, and to hospital administrators. Role clarification and positive outcomes are much more likely to guarantee CNSs a place in the future of health care.

Yes! The time *is* right for the next generation of CNSs to emerge and meet the challenges of health care reform. The profession of nursing has faced many changes and much evolution. Role evolution for CNSs is another transition that is required for nurses to meet the changing demands of health care. The success of CNSs making the transition will, in large part, depend upon nurse administrators facilitating, coordinating and integrating this role into the existing system.

REFERENCES

Allred, C. A., Arford, P. H., Michel, Y., Dring, R., Carter, V., & Vietch, J. S. (1995). A cost-effectiveness analysis of acute care case management outcomes. *Nursing Economics, 13(3),* 129-136.

American College of Physicians (1994). Physician Assistants and Nurse Practitioners. *Annals of Internal Medicine, 121(9),* 714-716.

Brockopp, D. Y., Porter, M., Kinnaird, S., & Silberman, S. (1992). Fiscal and clinical evaluation of patient care. *Journal of Nursing Administration, 22(9),* 23-27.

Brooten, D., Gennara, S., Knapp, H., Jovene, N., Brown, L., & York, R. (1991). CNS functions in early discharge of very low birthweight infants. *Clinical Nurse Specialist, 5,* 196-201.

Burge, S., Crigler, L., Hurt, L., Kelly, G., & Sanborn, C. (1989). Clinical nurse specialist role development: Quantifying actual practice over three years. *Clinical Nurse Specialist, 3(1),* 33-36.

Fenton, M. V. (1985). Identifying competencies of clinical nurse specialists. *Journal of Nursing Administration, 15,* 31-37.

Forbes, K. (1992). Live in the past . . . Or face the future??? *Clinical Nurse Specialist, 6(1),* 90.

Gillies, D. A. (1994). *Nursing management. A systems approach.* Philadelphia: W. B. Saunders.

Holt, F. M. (1987). Executive practice . . . developmental stages of the clinical nurse specialist role. *Clinical Nurse Specialist, 1(3),* 116-118.

Kennedy, L., Niedlinger, S., & Scroggins, K. (1987). Effective comprehensive discharge planning for hospitalized elderly. *The Gerontologist, 27,* 577-580.

Lynn-McHale, D. J., Fitzpatrick, E. R., & Shaffer, R. B. (1993). Case management: Development of a model. *Clinical Nurse Specialist, 7*(6), 299-307.

Minarik, P. A. (1990). Collaboration between service and education: Perils or pleasures for the clinical nurse specialist? *Clinical Nurse Specialist, 4*(2), 109-114.

Neidlinger, S., Scroggins, K., & Kennedy, L. (1987). Cost evaluation of discharge planning for hospitalized elderly. *Nursing Economics, 5*(5), 225-230.

Page, N. E., & Arena, D. M. (1994). Rethinking the merger of the clinical nurse specialist. *IMAGE, 26*(4), 315-318.

Simms, L. M., Price, S. A., & Ervin, M. E. (1994). *The professional practice of nursing administration.* Albany: Delmar.

Soehren, P. M., & Schumann, L. L. (1994). Enhanced role opportunities available to the CNS/nurse practitioner. *Clinical Nurse Specialist, 8*(3), 123-127.

South Carolina Nurse. (1994, Summer). Nursing's agenda for health care reform.

Sparacino, P. S. (1991). The CNS-case management relationship. *Clinical Nurse Specialist, 5*(4), 180-181.

Strong, A. G. (1992). Case management and the CNS. *Clinical Nurse Specialist, 6*(1), 64.

Tappen, R. M. (1995). *Nursing leadership and management. Concepts and practice.* Philadelphia: F. A. Davis.

Vestal, K. W. (1995). *Nursing management, concepts and issues.* Philadelphia: J. B. Lippincott.

Walker, M. (1986). How nursing service administrators view clinical nurse specialists. *Nursing Management, 16,* 31-36.

Wolf, G. A. (1990). Clinical nurse specialists: The second generation. *Journal of Nursing Administration, 20*(5), 7-8.

Yoder Wise, P. S. (1995). *Leading and managing in nursing.* St. Louis: Mosby.

CHAPTER 12

The Acute Care Nurse Practitioner: Innovative Practice for the 21st Century

Lisa Norsen
Ellen Fineout
Denise Fitzgerald
Deborah Horst
Rita Knight
Mary Ellen Kunz
Eileen Lumb
Beth Martin
Janice Opladen
Ellen Schmidt

The current health care environment supports the emergence of the acute care nurse practitioner (ACNP) as a necessary care provider who can address the increasingly complex needs of patients, hospital systems, insurers, and regulators. The ACNP is a sophisticated clinician who practices within a conceptual framework that articulates clearly the responsibilities of the role. The role is characterized by elements unique to advanced practice that position the ACNP to render comprehensive, cost-effective, efficient, and accessible care.

Profound changes in the health care system are inevitable and promise to create challenges for all nurses, especially for those practicing in acute care. This challenge requires innovative approaches to care delivery that ensure high-quality, cost-effective, and efficient practice models are in place. Advanced practice nurses (APNs) in acute care view the challenge as an opportunity to question the boundaries of traditional nursing and medical practice and to carve out new roles. The result has been the evolution of the acute care nurse practitioner (ACNP) role, an APN who promises not only to meet the demands of change, but also to provide leadership in shaping the future of nursing in the 21st century.

The purpose of this chapter is to describe the role of the ACNP as defined by an established Model of Advanced Practice, to demonstrate the contribution of the ACNP to practice and to examine some of the controversies that confront the ACNP in practice.

BACKGROUND

The history of the ACNP is rooted in the legacies of both the clinical nurse specialist (CNS) and the primary care nurse practitioner. The CNS and primary care nurse practitioner, as predecessors of the ACNP, developed their advanced practice domains in parallel fashion but with clear distinctions in temperament and direction. Although the roles of the CNS and the primary care nurse practitioner were both envisioned as a means to bring clinical expertise to defined populations, the focus of this expert care was different. Traditionally, the practice arena for the CNS was the tertiary care setting and focused on specialty patient populations, whereas the primary care nurse practitioner emerged as a direct care provider in the community emphasizing primary care services and health promotion. The responsibilities of the CNS in improving patient care were achieved primarily through the provision of indirect care services including role model, educator, consultant, and researcher (Elder & Bullough, 1990) as well as systems expert and change agent. Direct care responsibilities, although important to the role, were of secondary significance and usually highlighted psychosocial support for patients and families (Elder & Bullough, 1990). The primary care nurse practitioner has always emphasized provision of direct care dispensed via advanced assessments, therapeutics, and interventions. Traditional affiliations, though not absolute, have also differed: The CNS has been clearly aligned with nursing practice, and the primary care nurse practitioner has been more closely associated with medical practice.

IMPETUS FOR CHANGE

For many years, the differences in these two roles were considered strengths and each existed separately and successfully within their practice domains. In

more recent years, the boundaries distinguishing these roles became, by necessity, more blurred as trends in health care forced tertiary care facilities to
scrutinize their bureaucratic practices, reorganize hospital structures, and
prioritize institutional goals. In this environment, several factors influenced the
development of the acute care nurse practitioner role.

Advocates for quality care attacked the standard training routines for resident physicians. Specifically, the number of hours worked and the dangers
inherent in the system that promoted long hours and unsupervised decision
making were questioned. In New York State, the Ad Hoc Committee on
Emergency Services recommended constraints on the numbers of resident
hours worked and required closer monitoring of resident activities in an
attempt to ensure quality care (Bell, 1988). In addition, *The Study on Surgery
Services for the U.S.* advocated fewer resident positions to limit the number of
physicians in specialty practice (Gellhorn, 1988). This recommendation has
been fueled by health care reform initiatives that supported reallocation of
dollars for graduate medical education from specialty practice to primary care
to ensure basic universal coverage in the future (Safriet, 1992).

The high cost of delivering health care has prompted the government,
regulators, and insurers to examine how specialty care is provided. Factors
identified as contributing to high costs include the fragmentation and poor
coordination of care services, the relative inaccessibility of providers, and a
cumbersome and unresponsive care system. These factors combined with the
expected reduction in the availability of resident staff supported the emergence
of the ACNP, a new clinician who could combine the advanced skills of the
primary care nurse practitioner with the leadership, research, education, and
systems expertise of the Clinical Nurse Specialist.

MODEL OF ADVANCED PRACTICE FOR THE ACNP

The role of the ACNP is well established at the University of Rochester. The
first ACNP position was implemented in 1979 in cardiac surgery and has been
described elsewhere (Davitt & Jensen, 1981). Recently, the ACNP group in
surgical nursing practice developed a conceptual model to describe the unique
role of the ACNP. Practicing within a conceptual model is critical for success
as an ACNP. A model provides the structure necessary to define the appropriate
elements of advanced practice and, thus, a means to measure and guide it. A
model, when considered as an integrated whole, defines the commitment and
focus of advanced practice. Individual components of the model outline the
responsibilities and behaviors unique to advanced practice.

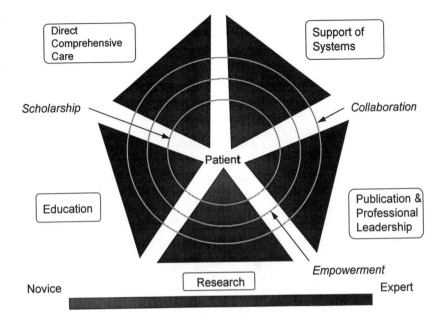

Figure 12.1: The Strong Model of Advanced Practice

Practical considerations warrant using a conceptual model at the advanced level. Economic constraints demand that all health care providers clearly articulate their contribution to quality patient care and evaluate outcomes. In addition, hospitals, insurers, regulators, and consumers are demanding that care providers address the increasingly complex problems of fragmented, disorganized, inaccessible, impersonal, and costly care. A well-defined model of practice is the structure on which these issues can be managed.

The Strong Model of Advanced Practice (Figure 12.1) was developed by Surgical Nursing Practice to organize practice accountabilities for ACNPs, to establish evaluative criteria for ACNPs and to negotiate collaborative responsibilities of ACNPs. The model is circular and includes five domains of practice that constitute its core elements: direct care, support of systems, education, research and publication, and professional leadership. The domains are considered to be mutually exclusive and described by unique behaviors exhaustive of role responsibilities (see Table 1). Enveloping the domains and providing unity to its structure are three conceptual strands: collaboration, empowerment, and scholarship. Collaboration is the balance of cooperation and assertiveness in decision making (Weis & Davis, 1985). Empowerment is the authority to make

TABLE 12.1   Examples of Domain Specific Behaviors

Direct Comprehensive Care:
   Consults and documents patient history and physical exam
   Identifies and initiates required diagnostic tests and procedures
   Performs specialty specific procedures

Support of System:
   Participates in strategic planning for the service, department, or hospital
   Provides leadership and actively participates in the assessment, development,
      implementation and evaluation of quality improvement programs

Research:
   Uses research and integrates theory into practice and recommends policy changes based
      on research
   Conducts clinical investigation
   Engineers/designs clinical information systems that make data available for future research

Education:
   Evaluates education programs and recommends revisions as needed
   Facilitates professional development of nursing staff through education

Publication and Professional Leadership:
   Serves as a resource or committee member in professional organizations
   Disseminates nursing knowledge through presentation or publication

---

decisions about practice issues, and scholarship is the constant inquiry about how and why decisions are made (Ackerman, Norsen, Martin, Wiedrich, Kitzman, 1996). These strands pervade the model and permeate each domain; thus, effective application of the model in the practice arena requires the synthesis of the three strands into each domain.

The patient and family form the foundation of the model and appear as its center. All components emanate from this core and the model only has meaning when it is applied within the context of patient and family. Elements and activities defined by the model are focused on providing excellent care.

A continuum of expertise lies at the base of the Strong Model and is premised on Benner's work (Benner, 1982). The continuum, from novice to expert, represents proficiency in executing behaviors describing the domains of practice and mastery in using conceptual strands in diverse situations. The continuum interacts continuously with the model and modifies the responsibilities of the ACNP within each domain according to his or her position on the spectrum.

Operationalizing the Model

Operationalization of the Strong Model assumes various forms and does not imply simultaneous implementation of all domains or infer concurrent expertise in each domain of practice. Also, implicit to implementation is an appreciation for its practice focus that requires that all behaviors are concentrated on achieving quality clinical outcomes.

The Strong Model is intended to be dynamic to meet the changing needs inherent in clinical practice. The ACNP negotiates involvement and responsibility in each domain according to service needs, professional experience and goals, and personal interest. Although it is desirable to renegotiate commitment to various domains periodically, an ACNP undertaking a new role initially negotiates primary responsibility in the domain of direct comprehensive care. Absolute commitment to this domain is necessary in the beginning to develop clinical expertise in specialty practice, validate collaborative relationships with clinical colleagues and establish role credibility. Once the role is well established, and the ACNP well acquainted with clinical practice, the other domains can be fully integrated.

The continuum of expertise determines the proficiency of the ACNP in performing the behaviors described within each domain. For example, in the domain direct care, the experienced ACNP is more proficient than the novice ACNP in conducting assessments, evaluating laboratory results and diagnostics, planning interventions, and would be considered expert in these behaviors. The ACNP can become expert in any or all behaviors characteristic of each domain, and the experience of the ACNP as well as the requirements of the position will determine which behaviors should be developed. For example, facilitating research and conducting research are both behaviors in the domain research. A newly appointed or experienced ACNP with limited research interest can collect data or contribute clinical insights regarding the conduct of an investigation and demonstrate proficiency in facilitating research in this manner. On the other hand, the senior ACNP may be managing independent clinical investigations expertly.

The conceptual strands characterize the approach or attitude of the ACNP in operationalizing the model. Any behavior articulated within the domains of practice is distinguished by scholarship, collaboration, and empowerment. The continuum of expertise describes the success of the ACNP in synthesizing these concepts into daily practice. For example, the novice ACNP, although empowered to implement practice changes as described in support of systems, may not have the skills (e.g., systems acumen, intraprofessional affiliations, personal knowledge) necessary to exercise empowerment. Likewise, a novice ACNP does not possess the professional sophistication to fully actualize collaboration and may be initially more "cooperative" than "assertive" in decision making. The experienced ACNP understands the symmetry of cooperation and assertiveness in achieving quality outcomes and is therefore an expert in collaboration.

When the Strong Model is fully operationalized, the ACNP is involved, to varying degrees, in every domain of practice. The ACNP always maintains a clinical focus that is rooted in the direct care of patients. ACNP practice, and by association, patient care, is buttressed by the clinician's involvement in system support, education, professional leadership, and research.

Although the experienced ACNP may be highly skilled in all behaviors and capable of demonstrating expertise in all domains, it is unrealistic to expect that an ACNP is equally involved and expert in all domains of practice simultaneously. It is not feasible to operationalize the model in this manner. If attempted, role responsibilities become unmanageable and the model becomes untenable. Individual ACNPs must negotiate role responsibilities and adjust commitment to individual domains according to professional goals and clinical or systems needs. This dynamic aspect of the model ensures that the role remains challenging and responsive to changing professional and clinical priorities.

INNOVATIVE AND EFFECTIVE PRACTICE

Understanding application of the model provides good insight about the role, but a true appreciation of the potential contribution of the ACNP to acute care requires an understanding of specific factors that distinguish advanced practice. The following factors are integral to advanced practice.

Direct Care

The direct care responsibilities of the ACNP are the foundation of advanced practice and challenge conventional wisdom that firmly established the physician as the only qualified purveyor of medical care. The ACNP consistently pushes the boundaries of practice accountability by determining medical diagnoses and prescribing medical and pharmacologic treatment interventions. In states with advanced practice laws, the ACNP is fully authorized to carry out and modify the medical plan of care, thus defining the expanded Scope of Practice and Standards of Practice unique to ACNPs. The expanded Scope of Practice is carried out within the boundaries of a collaborative practice arrangement, generally with physicians, and established practice protocols or practice guidelines (Norsen, Opladen, & Quinn, 1995). For example, the ACNP in the intensive care unit manages daily decision making about the progression of critically ill cardiac surgery patients through an accelerated postoperative care program. This progression is outlined according to practice protocols established for the patient population. The ACNP individualizes care according to ongoing assessments and, when necessary, modifications in the plan of care.

The ACNP provides direct care services within a specialty population and the focus of the care is determined by the ACNP and the collaborating physician. The spectrum of direct care spans the continuum of care, and the breadth of responsibilities assumed by the ACNP is impressive. Some have suggested that the ACNP can be used as a resident replacement (Silver & McAtee, 1988). Although it is true that the ACNP is capable of performing many of the services and skills traditionally associated with resident care, care rendered by the ACNP is unique, and by some measures, superior.

It has been well established that primary care nurse practitioners can provide care that is equal to and in some cases better than their physician counterparts (Ramsay, 1982; Salkever, 1982; Sox, 1979). This precept has not been tested in the acute care setting, but pioneers in the clinical arena have consistently demonstrated their proficiency in a wide range of skills. It is typical for ACNPs to be performing skills ranging from tube and line removal to invasive procedures such as femoral arterial line insertion, chest tube insertion, central line insertion, or anoscopy. The ACNP undergoes a credentialing process whereby competence in a broad range of skills is demonstrated (Table 12.2).

Characteristics of Advanced Practice

Several characteristics qualify the ACNP as unique. A distinguishing characteristic of ACNP care is the approach to delivery of care that assimilates both medical and nursing perspectives. This approach is pervasive in all interactions and encounters. Admission or intake procedures illustrate this blended role perspective. During the admission assessment, the ACNP conducts the history and physical concentrating on the regional or specialty exam (e.g., cardiac or orthopedic) specific to the presenting problem and incorporates a comprehensive screening exam that encompasses the precepts of health promotion and maintenance. In addition, functional and pyschosocial assessments are an integral component of the intake interview when conducted by the ACNP. This facilitates the identification and management of problems promptly and forms the basis for both the nursing and medical plans of care. Patient teaching, performed throughout the intake process, has a distinctive quality when done by the ACNP whose perspective combines both medical and nursing concerns. This encompassing perspective goes beyond patient care to the institutional level. The ACNP views all issues beyond the traditional delineations and is an advocate of creative change and reorganization of structures to accommodate redesigns that promote quality and cost efficiency. For example, the ACNP in general surgery redesigned the preoperative program for patients undergoing colon surgery. Through a screening procedure, selected patients are prepared for their surgery at home. This preparation includes both nursing and medical

TABLE 12.2 Credentialing Manual for ACNP (examples)

Arterial Puncture
    * Radial
    * Femoral

Chest Tube Management
    * Insertion
    * Removal
    * Plueroderis
    * Conversion into empyema tubes

Compartment Pressure Measurement

Intravenous Puncture and Line Insertion
    * Peripheral
    * Central

Temporary Pacemaker Wire Removal

Thoracentesis

Tracheostomy Tube Change
    * Fenestrated
    * Non-fenestrated
    * Metal

Traction Application/Manipulation
    * Bucks
    * Bryants
    * Russel
    * Split Russel
    * 90°—90°
    * Balanced Suspension
    * Cervical
    * Pelvic
    * Dunlops

Nasal Packing
    * Insertion
    * Removal

Wound Management
    * Aspiration
    * Culture
    * Debridement
    * Drain removal
    * Foreign body removal from subcutaneous site
    * Incision and drainage
    * Infiltration for administration of local anesthesia
    * Packing (including wick insertion)
    * Suturing—subcutaneous closure/cutaneous closure
    * Suture removal
    * Staple removal

considerations, such as education and bowel preparation, and has resulted in increased patient satisfaction and reduced length of stay.

Two essential components that discriminate ACNP practice are coordination of care and continuity of care. The ACNP is particularly capable of coordinating care for a specialty population. First, the ACNP is very familiar with established standards of care for the specialty population. The ACNP also possesses the savvy to manipulate the health care system for patient benefit and has the interpersonal skills and the professional credibility to communicate effectively within the interdisciplinary team. Finally, the ACNP has the necessary clinical skills to make advanced assessments and is authorized to implement changes in care as needed. The ACNP is a recognized practitioner who possesses the clinical authority and leadership capability necessary to competently coordinate and facilitate patient care. For example, discharge of the acutely ill patient is often a complex process. The ACNP facilitates the discharge process by performing the appropriate nursing and medical assessments to determine suitability for discharge. Once this determination is made, the ACNP garners the resources necessary to expedite discharge and provides ongoing medical and nursing support for the patient, family, and community care providers after discharge.

Continuity of care has two frameworks for the ACNP. In the first, the ACNP remains a "constant" in the interdisciplinary team and therefore provides continuity in care delivered from day to day, week to week, month to month, or even year to year. While resident staff and other members of the team rotate on and off service, the ACNP by his or her continuity, ensures that standards are maintained. The ACNP functions as a role model demonstrating "best practice" in the delivery of both medical and nursing care for the patient. In this context, coordination of care and continuity of care contribute not only to quality but also to reduced cost. The ACNP ensures adherence to established protocols that reduces redundancy of services, duplication of effort and overuse of limited resources.

The other aspect of continuity addresses the continuum of care where the ACNP follows the patient for the acute episode and then into the illness rehabilitation, chronicity, or remission. For example, in orthopedics, the ACNP on the spine team follows patients and families from the Emergency Department through the ICU, to the orthopedic unit, and into the inpatient and outpatient rehabilitation settings. This facet of care moves the patient with complex medical and psychosocial problems seamlessly through the system, ensuring adherence to an organized and efficient plan of care.

Commitment and professional maturity are important traits that the ACNP brings to practice. The ACNP, although a continuous learner, is not a student in the role as is the resident physician. The ACNP is committed to the patient and the institution and thus invested in the process and outcomes of care. This does not imply that residents do not give good patient care but, rather, that the focus of their endeavor is to learn. ACNPs are building a career and thus able to devote energy necessary to provide quality care. The domain, Support of Systems, probably illustrates this best with behaviors such as participating in strategic planning and quality improvement activities.

ACNPs are well versed in the importance of outcomes management and by temperament and experience are capable of providing leadership in the efforts to affect quality, cost effective, outcome-focused care. ACNPs are uniquely qualified to organize outcomes management because of their ability to combine clinical expertise with systems insights and leadership acumen. The ACNP is credible with clinical colleagues and administrators and therefore able to not only analyze the issues and ensure change but also elicit the support and "buy in" necessary for success.

Such versatility is illustrated by an ACNP who led an interdisciplinary team in addressing quality of care and length of stay for vascular surgery patients. The ACNP used a Total Quality Management framework to facilitate group process and recommend both medical and nursing practice changes. These changes were diverse, ranging from the introduction of care maps and the development of population specific flow sheets and patient education materials to the introduction of telemetry monitors on the surgical inpatient units. The work of this team resulted in decreased mean lengths of stay for four surgical DRG groups, saved significant health care dollars, and improved quality as measured by defined morbidities and in hospital mortalities.

ISSUES IN ADVANCED PRACTICE

Although the ACNP is capable of innovative and effective practice, success in the future will require thoughtful consideration and a thorough understanding of issues related to advanced practice. Several emergent role issues will be examined.

Collaborative Practice

As presented, the tenets of collaboration underlie successful advanced practice. A collaborative practice model for acute care has been described by Norsen, Opladen, and Quinn (1995) and is based on the premise that highly complex patients seen in the acute care setting cannot be managed by a single care provider but, rather, rely on the combined expertise of a cadre of health professionals. This collaborative practice model recognizes the unique contributions of physicians and the ACNPs to care and contends that there is limited overlap of expertise. Schematically, this has been illustrated as intersecting circles (King, Parrinello, & Baggs, in press).

For this dyad to work, the ACNP and MD must understand and participate in the collaborative process. Although the ACNP has a keen comprehension of collaboration, physicians have much less experience with collaborating with nurses. ACNP need to continue to promote collaboration and distinguish ACNP practice as desirable and unique. Many physicians view the ACNP as a physician extender and may consider the relationship as supervisory rather than collaborative. ACNP must be confident in their own abilities to render quality cost-effective care, to positively influence outcomes and ultimately to implement change. ACNP must also be politically astute and recognize the potential for competition among care providers as acute care services are re-engineered. With the framework, it is incumbent upon ACNPs to demonstrate their contribution to institutional initiatives and cost saving strategies.

Once strong collaborative relationships have been established, there is opportunity for the ACNP to institute independence within the collaborative framework in specified areas of interest. For example, the ACNPs in general surgery have instituted an ambulatory wound clinic. Although this clinic is maintained within the structure of the practice agreement written with the chairman of surgery, the ACNPs directly receive referrals for chronic wounds related to postoperative wound infections, venous stasis disease, small vessel disease, and pressure ulcers. They manage wounds over the long term and are directly responsible for the success of the clinic.

Role Differentiation

Contrasting the advanced practice roles of the ACNP and the CNS facilitates understanding the uniqueness of the ACNP role. Debate about role differentiation and role mergers between the nurse practitioner and the CNS has continued for more than 10 years (Page & Arena, 1994). Although the ACNP combines selected characteristics from both the primary care nurse practitioner and the CNS roles, the ACNP is not intended as a replacement for either one. The acute care structure requires the focused contribution of the CNS to nursing staff education and program initiatives, as well as the contribution of the ACNP to direct patient care issues for a specific population. The Strong Model of Advanced Practice supports both CNS and ACNP roles and provides a window through which the roles can be clarified and understood. When examined within the framework of the model, it is clear that each role has unique primary and secondary responsibilities within each of the five domains, which differentiates them, and shared responsibilities that unite them.

Primary and Secondary Roles

The CNS and the ACNP both have teaching responsibilities; however, their focus is different. The primary role of the CNS is focused on nursing education, staff orientation, and role development. Programs developed for individuals or groups of nursing staff can have a general or specialty focus. The CNS provides direct support of systems, assists staff to implement new procedures and products, and assesses the effectiveness of new processes on patient outcomes. The learners may be limited to a particular nursing specialty or encompass all nursing staff within the institution. The CNS plays a key role in the development of standards of care and protocols specific to a process or product.

The ACNP's primary focus is directing and participating in comprehensive patient care. The role provides nursing linkages to the interdisciplinary team in assessing, prescribing, and defining the required interventions. The ACNP role is directed toward the individual patient or specialty group, and addresses the immediate and ongoing care needs of this group of patients.

The primary ACNP role of direct care is a secondary role of the CNS. CNS, in collaboration with the nursing staff and health care team, are involved in one-on-one patient and staff consultation that is problem focused. Their direct care linkages include developing care maps, assessing patient care outcome variances, and creating approaches to address and resolve systems issues influencing the effectiveness or timeliness of patient care.

The primary CNS role of education and systems support is a secondary role for the ACNP. The direct care nature of the ACNP role allows the practitioner to take advantage of the window of opportunity for learning. This often takes the form of "just-in-time" teaching patients about their relevant issues or concerns. The ACNP's role in clinical problem-solving is a collaborative effort with staff and is related to specific patient populations.

The ACNP is involved in both staff education and support of systems as issues affect a specific patient population. The primary forum for ACNPs to address system concerns related to their specialty population is total quality management (TQM) teams that deal with a specific problem or process. The CNS perspective on systems issues is more global and comprehensive.

The CNS and ACNP roles offer perspectives on the same issues. The roles complement one another and provide a more comprehensive approach to patient care management. The involvement of both the CNS and ACNP in consultation and problem-solving provides more extensive resources to determine and facilitate the best intervention and management for a given patient situation.

Shared Responsibilities

Both the ACNP and the CNS have shared scholarly responsibilities in research, publication, and professional leadership. The CNS has a system focus and the ACNP has a patient care focus, with their common ground enhanced by their collaboration with each other and the health care team. Both roles encompass formal education programs and scholarly research as well as collaboration in seminars, conferences, and academic and continuing education presentations.

CNS involvement in quality improvement (QI) and TQM problem-solving teams is directed toward general system changes such as development of mechanical prevention standards for deep vein thrombosis, and evaluation and introduction of patient controlled analgesia therapy. The ACNP is involved in specialty-based problem-solving teams around issues such as addressing length of stay and revising patient care interventions and protocols. The CNS and ACNP often collaborate to accomplish joint projects such as devising a system for tracking equipment use and availability and facilitating retrieval of equipment to more readily meet patient needs.

Both roles expand beyond QI to formal research protocols. The CNS focuses on evaluation and implementation of system changes such as the introduction of cross-trained technicians. The ACNP focuses on research efforts toward specific patient populations such as the evaluation of the use of a foley catheter versus straight catheterization in the postoperative patient. Both inquiries can have a direct bearing on patient care, while incorporating interdisciplinary problem-solving. There are many opportunities for collaborative research among ACNPs and CNSs that address specific patient issues across different patient populations. These partnerships result in a comprehensive approach to meeting both patient and staff needs. Optimization of these roles involves recognizing the strengths of each position and then determining the correct mix of ACNPs and CNSs to accomplish strategic goals.

Organizational Structure

For ACNP practice to be successful, several organizational issues must be addressed. The hospital bureaucracy is notorious for its cumbersome rules and sluggish approaches to change. These characteristics are inconsistent with the Strong Model and the vision for health care in the 21st century which rely on empowerment, collaboration, accountability, and innovation. Therefore, for the ACNP to be successful, the typical hierarchical and bureaucratic system must be replaced with a structure where clinicians are responsible for decisions affecting their practice. In the future, the traditional institutional hierarchies must be replaced by program initiatives that rely on collaborative nursing, physician, and administrative alliances to direct care and which are evaluated by defined quality indicators. In this structure, the ACNP role is defined by the Scope of Practice for advanced practice and collaborative with other clinicians and administrators so that the outcome reflects economic as well as clinical realities. Within this framework, practitioners must be empowered to implement change quickly and, thus, remain responsive to the constantly changing needs of the patient and the system.

Three organizational models exist for ACNP practice (El-Sherit, 1995). In the physician group practice model, the ACNP joins a physician practice and is affiliated with the hospital only by practice privileges and not at all to nursing. This model provides economic benefits for both the ACNP and the hospital because the ACNP shares in the profits of the practice and the hospital does not pay for services rendered. There are overriding disadvantages, however, because the ACNP is often isolated from nursing colleagues, thus loosing credibility as a nurse (Parrinello, 1995), and is viewed essentially as a physician extender. This dilutes the effectiveness of the ACNP in linking medical and nursing practice.

For years CNSs have operated successfully as practitioners in the nursing-based model. In this model, the CNS is hired by nursing, responsible solely to nursing administration and is assigned to a practice area to address specific clinical issues (Parrinello, 1995). Although there is no ambiguity regarding the focus or alliance in this design, it is fraught with problems for the ACNP. The lines that separate the medical and nursing practices have intentionally blurred as ACNPs have assumed many of the functions previously carried out exclusively by physicians. The nursing-based model encourages distinctions that have little relevance. Although it is absolutely vital that ACNPs retain their nursing identity, it is counterproductive to consider the role as separate from medical practice. There is also economic danger in subscribing to the nursing model for ACNPs. In this model, salaries are often subsumed within the nursing budget, which is often the largest expenditure in the hospital. As administrators begin scrutinizing budgets, ACNP positions might be at risk.

The third and most desirable model is the joint-practice model in which the ACNP-MD dyad forms the basis for a collaborative undertaking. This model recognizes the complementary roles of the two clinicians in delivering comprehensive, quality care. This model is the most complex model because its matrix structure produces alliances for the ACNP within both nursing and medicine.

Traditionally, this has created tension for the ACNP who has conflicts about loyalty, responsibility, and accountability. This confusion, however, is not necessary if the model works as intended. That is, the ACNP practices in a flattened organizational structure where collaboration replaces supervision and the role of the ACNP remains anchored in nursing practice but irrevocably linked to medicine. Although the collaborative joint practice model holds the most promise for ACNPs, it must be operationalized carefully and several professional issues should be considered.

Reporting Structure

In the collaborative joint-practice model, traditional reporting structures are replaced with individual accountability. The ACNP take responsibility for practice by demonstrating accountability for outcome measures important to nursing practice, physician colleagues, and the hospital. The outcomes are determined through collaboration and can include patient-focused outcomes (e.g., satisfaction), systems-focused outcomes (e.g., length of stay) or practitioner-focused outcomes (e.g., volume indicators). The ACNP cannot be solely responsible for each of these outcomes, and an important task of the collaborative joint practice is shared responsibility for outcomes.

Evaluation

Traditionally, ACNPs in joint practice models have reported to physicians for performance evaluations in clinical practice areas and nursing in areas such as program development, systems improvement, and professional practice (Parrinello, 1995). This fragmented approach to performance appraisal is based on the premise that physicians have little knowledge about nursing issues and vice versa. Ideally, the ACNP should undergo self- and peer evaluations with input from the collaborating physicians and nurses. An experienced ACNP should be responsible for coordinating the evaluations for a group of ACNPs with similar clinical responsibilities. This ensures consistency, comparability, and objectivity in the process. The structure for the evaluation can be based on the Strong Model and relies on the domains to define elements of the evaluation and the continuum of expertise to determine mastery. This does not imply that a new ACNP focusing on the direct care domain cannot receive an excellent evaluation or that a seasoned ACNP must be expert in each domain. Rather, negotiated responsibilities are accomplished.

Structure of Practice

As the ACNP role continues to develop, it is necessary to clarify role responsibilities and professional relationships within the structure of a practice agreement. Without the formality of this definition, the role can easily become untenable for the ACNP and unjustifiable for the administrator.

Before a meaningful practice agreement can be negotiated, the ACNP must acknowledge the role as a professional enterprise requiring flexibility beyond the constraints of the traditional work week and adaptability to accept the challenges of an evolving, dynamic role. The ACNP must be cognizant of appropriate boundaries around clinical practice. That is, the ACNP must be in control of the direction and focus of the role, thus avoiding misunderstandings and miscues about role expectation. For example, the ACNP is being regarded in many quarters as a resident replacement. This perspective does a grave injustice to the role and releases the specialty care resident from valuable learning experiences.

With a clear vision of advanced practice, the ACNP negotiates a practice agreement with both nursing and physician colleagues to address professional practice requirements, call responsibility, coverage for absences within the collaborative practice, patient population being served, methods for defining division of labor and responsibility, mechanisms for conflict resolution, professional (nonclinical) time, educational opportunities, mechanisms for communication and a reporting structure, and support services such as computer access and secretarial support.

A necessary complement to the practice agreement is an explicit Scope of Practice and Standards of Practice. A joint effort by the American Nurses' Association and the American Association of Critical Care Nurses recently published a Scope and Standards for ACNPs that should be adopted by all practitioners (ANA Publication, 1995). In addition, a credentialing and privileging process must be established to ensure that the ACNP has the skills and expertise required to practice safely (Smith, 1993). Credentialing provides the mechanism to document professional and technical competencies within the ACNP defined Scope of Practice. In the joint practice model, the process is initiated by the ACNP and reviewed by both collaborating nurses and physicians with a single recommendation granting privileges. This mechanism provides a safeguard for the ACNP, the institution, and the collaborating physician.

As positions within the health care system are scrutinized, professional productivity will be vital in securing role visibility. The ACNP must therefore develop a system to record activity. This can be accomplished in a variety of ways but must document contributions to institutional goals, progress toward personal goals, and demonstrate cost efficiency. Certification of productivity can be structured around the domains of practice and articulated using the domain-specific behaviors. For example, the direct care domain can be represented as volume indicators such as the number of admissions performed or consultation requests received, research in progress or clinical investigations, and support of system by leadership in implementing change.

Economics

Currently, no standards exist regarding equitable pay for ACNP. There is published information about salary for NP in primary care showing great variability depending on area and type of practice. This information probably does not translate easily into the acute care setting, however, because of differences in the models of delivery and role responsibility. There is debate regarding how to compensate ACNP. The controversy centers around the higher costs associated with employing ACNP when compared to resident staff. This argument is based on resident staff working longer hours for less pay. The argument is erroneous because it ignores the contribution of the ACNP in lowering overall health costs by providing continuity of care and coordinating services while maintaining or even increasing caseload.

ACNP salaries should be derived from both hospital and private practice accounts. The necessity of obtaining support from physician accounts may provoke some ACNPs because it infers a supervisory tenor to the collaborative relationship. The fact remains, however, that ACNPs contribute to increased revenue in private practice by increased volume of patients seen or services rendered. In the acute care setting, this reality must be reconciled in dollars and underscores the need for ACNPs to track and document contributions and negotiate salaries or profit sharing accordingly.

Currently, there is no reimbursement mechanism for the professional services provided by the ACNP and their contributions to care are bundled under hospital admission fees. There has been significant debate over the ACNP's right to receive third-party reimbursement for services, particularly for procedures traditionally performed by physicians. This issue is rapidly becoming irrelevant as the future of health care suggests the advent of a capitated system where there is no distinction between provider and hospital components of care. In a capitated plan, a contract is forged between an interested group (insurer or corporation) and a health care system that is given a predetermined amount of money to provide services. This fixed income is divided among all the providers of care and the hospital, all of whom share responsibility for efficient, safe, and cost-effective care. Reimbursement issues for ACNPs in a capitated system shift to substantiating contribution to patient care and then negotiating for "a piece of the pie." In the capitated system, the ACNP is an attractive option who adds significantly to the achievement of positive patient outcomes. The ACNP, who has already demonstrated capitated as an affordable, versatile, and innovative care provider is in a unique position to capitalize on the changes and challenges of the future.

SUMMARY

The ACNP is a new care provider who is uniquely qualified to provide efficient, effective care in the 21st century. The ACNP possesses the skills required to meet the ever-increasing demands of the acutely ill patient in the redesigned health care system. The ACNP is a flexible care provider who easily traverses the boundaries of medical and nursing practice to render comprehensive services.

The role of the ACNP is defined by the Strong Model of Advanced Practice, which describes the domains of practice as direct comprehensive care, support of system, publication and professional leadership, research, and education. ACNPs negotiate clinical responsibilities within each domain to fulfill personal, practice, and systems priorities. The model is fluid and capable of adaptation as the role and the health care system continues to evolve.

The ACNP provides innovative practice perspectives through the provision of direct care services, care coordination, continuity of care, and outcomes management. Collaborative practice models must develop to address the issues and controversies that face the ACNP in the 21st century. Within this structure, a balance between professional autonomy and interdisciplinary dependence will establish the ACNP as an indispensable care provider.

REFERENCES

Ackerman, M., Norsen, L., Martin, B., Wiedrich, J., & Kitzman, H. (1996). The Strong model of advanced practice. *American Journal of Critical Care, 5*(1).

ANA Publication: Standards of Clinical Practice and Scope of Practice for the Acute Care Nurse Practitioner. (1995). Washington, DC: American Nurse Publishing.

Bell, B. (1995). The new hospital code and the supervision of residents. *NYS Journal of Medicine, 88*(12), 617-619.

Benner, P. (1982). From novice to expert. *American Journal of Nursing, 82*, 402-407.

Davitt, P., & Jensen, L. (1981, Fall). The role of the acute care nurse practitioner in cardiac surgery. *Nursing Administration Quarterly*, 16-19.

El-Scherif, C. (1995). Nurse practitioners—Where do they belong in within the organizational structure of the acute care setting? *Nurse Practitioner, 20*(1), 62-65.

Elder, and Bullough (1990). Nurse practitioners and clinical nurse specialists: Are the roles merging? *Clinical Nurse Specialist, 4*(2), 78-84.

Gellhorn, A. (1988). Recommendations on supervision and working conditions of residents. *NYS Journal of Medicine, 88*(1), 37.

King, K., Parrinello, K., & Baggs, J. (in press). Collaboration and collaborative models of practice. In J. Hickey, R. Ouimette, and S. Vengoni (Eds.), *Nurse Practitioners: Moving into the 21st Century*. Philadelphia: J. B. Lippincott.

Norsen, L., Opladen, J., & Quinn, J. (1995). Practice model: Collaborative practice. *Critical Care Nursing Clinics of North America, 7*(1), 43-52.

Page, N., & Arena, D. (1994). Rethinking the merger of the clinical nurse specialist and the nurse practitioner roles. *Image, 26*(4), 315-318.

Parrinello, K. (1995). Advanced practice nursing: An administrative perspective. *Critical Care Nursing Clinics of North America, 7*(1), 1-8.

Ramsay, J., McKenzie, J., & Fist, D. (1982). Physicians and nurse practitioners: Do they provide equivalent health care? *American Journal of Public Health, 72,* 142-153.

Safriet, B. J. (1992). Health care dollars and regulatory sense: The role of advanced practice nursing. *Yale Journal of Regulation, 9,* 419-488.

Silver, H., & McAtee, P. (1988). Should nurses substitute for house staff? *American Journal of Nursing, 88,* 1671-1673.

Smith, T. (1991). Structured process to credential nurses with advanced practice skills. *Journal of Nursing Quality Assurance, 5*(3), 40-57.

Sox, H. (1979). Quality of patient care by nurse practitioners and physician assistants: A ten year perspective. *Annals of Internal Medicine, 91,* 459-468.

Weiss, S., & Davis, H. (1985). Validity and reliability of the collaborative practice scales. *Nursing Research, 34,* 299-305.

CHAPTER 13

Complementarity of Advanced Practice Nursing Roles in Enhancing Health Outcomes of the Chronically Ill: Acute Care Nurse Practitioners and Nurse Case Managers

Mary K. Walker
Juliann G. Sebastian

This chapter describes two evolving roles in which advanced practice nurses provide complementary services to chronically ill populations. We describe the clinical and system needs of chronically ill individuals and their families or other caregivers, then focus both on the content of the roles of acute care nurse practitioners and nurse case managers and on the complementarity of these roles. Collaboration between advanced practice nurses holds great potential for enhancing the health outcomes of populations requiring multiple, complex health and social services spanning long periods of time, such as those who are chronically ill. Operationalizing the complementarity of the roles of acute care nurse practitioners and nurse case managers makes it possible to provide seamless care for clients both within the context of a single episode of illness and across a continuum of care. This chapter describes these roles, their potential for complementary relationships, and their capacity for improving clinical and service utilization outcomes for chronically ill populations.

Reform of the health care system, particularly economic reform, has generated significant debate about issues fundamental to the delivery of health services. Among the issues receiving global attention are the financing of health services, the nature, structure, and composition of the health care workforce, the regulation of the health professions, and the potential for providing substantial patient benefits within an environment of significantly constrained resources.

The changes occurring in systems of care throughout the United States have led to increased attention to patients' needs for continuity of care and an emphasis on health rather than disease (Pew Health Professions Commission, 1995). In response to economic constraints and concerns about clinical outcomes that depend on effective functioning within service delivery networks, *seamless integration* is one goal of all health care systems. Seamless integration refers to providing health promotion and illness prevention services, caring for individuals across episodes of acute illness, managing transitions among settings in which care is delivered, and guiding individuals through the experiences associated with lifelong changes in health status.

This goal is important from a philosophical perspective because it is consistent with professional values and standards of practice, yet is responsive to the fiscal environment of health care. Consumers expect seamlessness as an indicator of service quality. Seamless clinical integration is also increasingly important in managed care arenas, because achieving effective clinical integration should reduce service fragmentation, more effectively help people maintain health, and reduce the need for more costly health services. This is especially desirable for integration efforts targeted toward populations most likely to require multiple, complex services spanning a long period of time, such as those who are chronically ill. Achieving the goal of seamless clinical integration requires new organizational processes and increased attention to personal and family health-related experiences throughout life.

Advanced practice nurses possess the skills needed to foster seamless integration in unique ways. Advanced practice nurses can provide comprehensive

AUTHORS' NOTE: This work was supported in part by the Bureau for Health Professions, Division of Nursing, Grant No. 1 D23 NU01186-01. The authors gratefully acknowledge the impact of discussions with faculty colleagues in both the Adult Nursing and the Community Health Nursing and Administration Divisions at the University of Kentucky College of Nursing and with the nurse consultants for this training grant. The thoughtful and penetrating questions of these colleagues have served to sharpen the ideas presented in this paper. The authors also wish to thank two anonymous reviewers whose insightful comments led to improvement in, and clarification of, the arguments in this chapter.

assessment of complex clinical needs of individuals and families, and they can place clinical needs within the context of socioeconomic and cultural factors within the community. They are expert clinicians and are able to diagnose, treat, and evaluate individual and family responses to clinical interventions. Advanced practice nurses increasingly are developing an understanding of the interactions between organizational, financial, and political environments within which health services are delivered and clinical and financial outcomes are realized. Because of this, they are well suited to developing population-based clinical programs that target the special needs of certain high-risk populations.

Reordering health care delivery into integrated systems predicts that different *types* of advanced practice nurses, as well as different *relationships* among these advanced practice providers, are required to achieve seamless integration. These new roles and relationships are essential regardless of whether service integration occurs within vertically integrated systems, such as full-scope, group practice health maintenance organizations, or whether such integration results from cooperation between autonomous health care agencies. Although much discussion has taken place around the need for effective interdisciplinary collaboration (cf., Pew Health Professions Commission, 1995), little dialogue has occurred about the benefits of collaborative *intradisciplinary* relationships on behalf of individuals and families over time. This chapter describes how the advanced practice nursing roles of acute care nurse practitioners and nurse case managers are evolving to provide complementary care for populations of chronically ill individuals and their families, facilitate seamless continuity of care, and contribute to achieving positive clinical and fiscal outcomes.

CLINICAL AND SYSTEM NEEDS OF
CHRONICALLY ILL POPULATIONS

The need for, and development of, these evolving advanced practice nursing roles is based in the special needs of chronically ill individuals and their families. All things being equal, chronically ill individuals and their families or other caregivers are more *vulnerable* to poor clinical outcomes than others (Aday, 1993). This means that they are both more sensitive to risk factors with which they may come into contact (Sebastian, 1996), and that their overall relative risk is greater than others because of interactions between their physiologic, psychologic, and social resources with risk factors (Aday, 1993). Vulnerability suggests that they risk not only exacerbations of their primary chronic illness and any comorbidities they may possess, but also that they are at higher risk than their healthier counterparts of developing new problems.

Risk for chronically ill individuals and their families can originate in: (1) physiologic and psychological limitations, (2) self-care demands, or (3) self-care agencies. One component of risk originates in physiologic vulnerabilities created by the individual's primary chronic illness. Another large component of risk arises out of the self-care demands placed both on the chronically ill individual and on those who care for or assist that person. By definition, chronically ill individuals possess ongoing therapeutic self-care needs (Orem, 1985) that consume time and energy. Therapeutic self-care demands can deflect an individual's time and energy away from other health promotion and illness prevention activities while they are engaged in the challenges associated with chronicity. Furthermore, therapeutic needs often precipitate lifestyle changes and require adaptation to new symptoms and acquisition of symptom management strategies. Such symptoms and symptom management strategies can, in and of themselves, contribute to psychosocial difficulties as the individual adapts to chronicity (Corbin & Strauss, 1988).

Another component of risk is associated with the extent to which chronically ill individuals and their families can assume self-care agency. Chronically ill individuals may infer that the health care system is equipped to provide for the majority of their needs, whereas health care professionals assume that those who are chronically ill will manage the majority of their self-care as well as uncomplicated episodes of illness associated with their diseases (Baker & Stern, 1993; Van Agthoven & Plomp, 1989). Mismatched beliefs such as these are likely to reduce the chronically ill individual's self-care effectiveness and satisfaction with services and the system's capacity to accommodate the health care requirements of these individuals.

Family and significant others often provide significant care and support for chronically ill individuals. Aday (1993, 1994) concluded that social resources are one key variable related to overall risk. Sebastian (1996) argued that social isolation and disenfranchisement reinforce the cycle of risk and the potential for poor outcomes. Family care, however, can create problems for family members and alter family dynamics, because of limited family resources, such as time, psychic and physical energy, money, and needs for respite. Unfortunately, the time costs and care requirements are essentially invisible in the current environment, thus compounding the sense of isolation and burden.

Chronically ill individuals have needs related to preventing exacerbations of illnesses, managing symptoms, and maintaining or improving their functional status and quality of life. In their grounded theory study of chronically ill individuals, Baker and Stern (1993) found that these individuals need to find meaning in their illnesses and develop a sense of control to be able to effectively manage their self-care needs. Of course, chronically ill individuals do experience acute exacerbations of their illnesses from time to time. At these times, they require expert nursing care to reduce the intensity of the exacerbation and the sequelae that can result. Family and caregiver clinical needs relate to perceived burdens associated with providing a wide range of supports for the chronically ill individual. These also can be categorized as physical, psychological, and social requirements. Such needs are related to fatigue, sleep deprivation, anxiety, social isolation of caregivers, potential resentment and anger, and knowledge deficits.

Chronically ill individuals and their families also possess needs related to systems of care because they typically require services from a wide variety of agencies to meet their diverse concerns (Provan & Milward, 1991). Whether such individuals receive services from vertically or horizontally integrated systems, the key challenge to providing a seamless experience is clinical integration (Lumsdon, 1994). From a system perspective, patients need assistance with identifying agencies that provide the services that would be helpful to them. They do not simply need service brokers, however. Rather, they truly need care coordinators. They need help identifying agencies that can provide a comprehensive service bundle and assistance to maximize referrals to multiple agencies, thus decreasing fatigue and frustration associated with working with multiple agencies (Sebastian, 1996). Such individuals may need an advocate to assemble the optimal configuration of services and negotiate favorable conditions, including insurance coverage, for receipt of services. Nurses are ideal providers to step into care coordinator roles. Advanced practice nurses have the skills to provide care coordination within and across settings, and to provide complex direct care as well to individuals and families. In particular, the complementary care that can be provided by acute care nurse practitioners and nurse case managers to chronically ill individuals and their families is likely to lead to improved health outcomes for, and efficient service use by, these populations.

COMPOSITION OF EVOLVING ROLES

Acute Care Nurse Practitioners

Much has been written about the roles of advanced practice primary care nurses and the equivalence of care delivered by these providers with services provided by physicians (Brown & Grimes, 1993; Office of Technology Assessment, 1986). A new category of care provider has emerged in high-intensity environments, both as a natural extension of the effectiveness of primary care nurse practitioners and as an evolution of the roles of acute care clinical nurse specialists (J. M. Clochesy, personal communication, August, 1995). These individuals are usually referred to as acute care nurse practitioners (ACNPs). Acute care nurse practitioners pursue advanced theoretical and practice knowledge consistent with their counterparts in other advanced practice programs. A clear distinction of the role of this emerging category of provider, however, is the inclusion of tasks commonly associated with the practice of medicine (Safreit, 1992). These expanded capabilities include the entire range of patient care delivery and surveillance of care; that is, options that can be exercised across the full continuum of acute care services.

The advanced practice role of ACNPs includes (1) management of acutely ill individuals throughout the entire episode of acute illness, (2) diagnosis of predictable deviations in the course of illness, (3) provision of ambulatory services in the acute transitional period following discharge (4) prescription of pharmacotherapeutics, and, (5) monitoring of drug and treatment efficacy (American Nurses Association, 1995b). These essential elements of advanced practice nursing in high intensity environments are provided in collaboration with other members of the health care team.

Developed as one response to fragmentation of services in the highly technological and specialty-oriented environments of acute care settings (American Nurses Association, 1995b), ACNPs have risen to national prominence, even as the profession has faced the challenge of reframing the delivery of high intensity patient care services (American Nurses Association, 1994).

The three key elements that have fueled development of the ACNP role are (1) access to care issues, (2) the aging of the American population, and (3) the contributions of chronicity and vulnerability to poor patient outcomes. The Standards of Clinical Practice and Scope of Practice for the Acute Care Nurse Practitioner expressed these realities clearly:

> Significant resources are expended for care that is specialty focused, often to the detriment of the continuity needs of patients in these settings. The result is an environment of high resource utilization and poorly configured patient outcomes. Furthermore, there is a mismatch among provider types, provider characteristics, and actual patient. . . . (American Nurses Association, 1995b, p. 10)

Stabilization and restoration of physical, psychological, and functional health status for acutely ill, highly unstable, and critically compromised individuals are the desired outcomes of care rendered by ACNPs. Major differences in role, however, preclude their being used interchangeably with clinical nurse specialists. For example, ACNPs, though nurses, have been substituted in some vertically integrated health care systems (e.g., Johns Hopkins) for house staff officers, just as family nurse practitioners have been substituted for primary care physicians in primary care settings. The practice of these nurses is characterized by expert clinical judgment across the full range of high-intensity services and accountability and authority for patient outcomes. The practice is always collaborative rather than independent, however (Clochesy, Daly, Idemoto, Steel, & Fitzpatrick, 1994). Further, their clinical decision making focuses on the specialty characteristics of the individuals who constitute their caseloads.

The specialty characteristics of individuals comprising the clinical caseloads of ACNPs actually drive both the preparation and the subsequent practice of these high-intensity advanced practice nurses. Because a preponderance of individuals requiring high-intensity nursing services are also chronically ill, the intensity and acuity of symptoms becomes an integral piece of the complexity of patient management. Further, symptom intensity as well as frequency and duration of symptom presentation, symptom number, and individual distress associated with symptoms (Lenz, Suppe, Gift, Pugh, & Milligan, 1995) affect the estimation or measurement of the intensity of nursing care requirements. Indeed, symptom presentation and intensity vary as much by contextual elements of symptom presentation (culture, ethnicity, gender, and age), psychological status (depression, anxiety, etc.), and functional capability (e.g., mobility), as by pathology and disease progression. Despite this, an emerging literature in nursing is attempting to examine the commonalities of symptom presentation across disease states and categories to delineate specific interventions and further explain the relationships between nursing interventions and patient outcomes.

A key feature, then, of the practice of ACNPs is that their practice is focused on patients' needs and is not bound to a particular setting. Although most ACNPs are currently employed by acute care facilities and likely spend the majority of their time practicing in these agencies, the role is evolving to one that is centered on the intensity of patient requirements and not the environment in which care is delivered. It is quite likely that much of high-intensity care may actually not occur in "hospitals" at all, but may occur in alternative settings such as long-term care, subacute units, ambulatory care, clinics, and the home. Given the predictions that managed care penetration will reach 80% to 90% in most U.S. markets and that as many as 50% of hospitals are likely to close by the year 2000 (Pew Health Professions Commission, 1995), it is especially likely that the setting of care will become less relevant to the practice of ACNPs than patient and family caregiver needs. Thus, in configuring ACNP roles, it is critical to both patient and organizational outcomes that these practitioners not be geographically limited. Rather, the practice of the ACNP "nurse intensivists" is configured on the basis of the specialty requirements of the patients for whom they are caring.

Further, the intervention strategies that ACNPs can use to manage symptoms include, but are not limited to, pharmacotherapy and the prescription of other traditional approaches, such as occupational therapy and physical therapy, to the high-acuity needs of chronically ill persons. Indeed, the intervention strategies are projected to incorporate the burgeoning nursing literature that embraces such diverse interventions as biofeedback, hypnosis, distraction, relaxation, and guided imagery (AHCPR, 1994; NINR, 1994). ACNPs collaborate with other providers in the delivery of these interventions over time. For example, as chronically ill patients make the transition from acute exacerbation to recovery and to managing the work of living with chronic illness, nurse case managers resume the role of providing long-term nursing to these individuals.

Nurse Case Managers

Nurse case managers (NCMs) assume roles as direct care providers, service coordinators, client advocates, family teachers, and system gatekeepers (Bower, 1992). As used in this chapter, the term "nurse case manager" refers to an evolution of, and convergence between the roles of nurse case managers, clinical nurse specialists, and primary care nurse practitioners. This evolution began with the work public health nurses pioneered around the turn of the century.

Nurses have provided professional case management services throughout the history of the profession. The concept of case management originated in Lillian Wald's work at the Henry Street Settlement House in New York City at the turn of the 20th century (Lancaster, 1996). Wald's concepts of long-term commitment to a particular community, becoming enmeshed in community life, and recognizing the interaction between health and social needs formed the basis for both public health nursing and social work. Throughout much of this century, public health nurses and social workers have functioned as case managers and have developed a variety of models of community-based case management (Bower, 1992).

Nurse case management in acute care settings developed throughout the 1980s, largely as an expansion of primary nursing, and later as an evolution of the role of acute care clinical nurse specialists (Cohen & Cesta, 1993; Zander, 1988). Goals normally include provision of high-quality, appropriate services and minimization of the length of stay for high-volume, high-risk, problem prone patient populations. Nurse case managers in acute care settings report improved clinical outcomes, enhanced patient satisfaction, and reductions in service utilization and cost (cf., Ethridge, 1991; Ethridge & Lamb, 1989). The distinction between nursing case management practiced within acute care settings and that which is based in the community has been termed "within the walls" and "beyond the walls," respectively (Cohen & Cesta, 1993). Nurse case managers are now linking care across settings in continuum-based models. The Nursing HMO at Carondelet St. Mary's in Tucson is a well-known example (Lamb & Huggins, 1990).

In addition to nurse case managers, individuals with a wide range of backgrounds have been employed as case managers, most commonly by managed care organizations and workers' compensation programs. This plethora of credentials in case management has made it difficult to differentiate the contributions of individuals with varying levels of preparation. Case managers of all types provide some direct services, particularly in systems with limited resources (Sebastian, 1994). Only nurse case managers provide direct clinical services, however. Within nursing, individuals with AD, BSN, and MSN preparation function as case managers (Lancero & Gerber, 1995). The nursing profession has not yet differentiated the contributions of those with differing levels of preparation, although Lamb (1995) challenges nursing to differentiate its contributions from those of others. Furthermore, the Pew Health Professions Commission (1995) recommends that baccalaureate prepared nurses provide care management within hospitals. In this chapter, we argue that advanced practice nurses are uniquely prepared to provide population-focused case management within and across systems.

As defined here, an advanced practice nurse case manager is an evolving role that begins with epidemiologic assessment of the needs of high-risk target populations and includes provision of direct care services in the form of individual and family assessment, care planning, care delivery, monitoring, and evaluation across settings and over time. Thus, nurse case managers provide distributive care (Lysaught, 1970, cited in Hall & Weaver, 1977) focused on assisting individuals and families with long-term health problems. The NCM's emphasis is on client advocacy within explicit organizational constraints. Organizational constraints include the financial constraints posed by reimbursement policies and managed care realities of cost control, as well as service constraints arising out of the service configuration within individual agencies and across the range of services available within a local community. The direct care role functions are in addition to brokering and coordinating the multiple services often needed by chronically ill individuals and their families. We propose that role expansion of either community-based or acute care nurse case management is necessary to achieve full continuity of care for chronically ill populations. The shifts in the health care system toward more formally integrated service delivery systems and managed care arrangements not only provide the organizational arrangements that support a continuum-based model of nursing case management, but that also demand that each health professional provide the full range of health services consistent with their professional capability.

The evolution of the role is toward assisting individuals and families manage the care that is necessary to both promote health and prevent illness, irrespective of the site of care delivery. The emphasis on care allows advanced practice nurses to distinguish the focus of their work from that of non-nurse case managers. In addition, this reflects a more population-based orientation; that is, toward care of selected target populations, and an orientation toward families and other caregivers, as compared with an individualistic orientation. This emphasis reflects the beneficial nature of the clinical outcomes that nurse case managers have been achieving over past years, and places attention on clinical care, whether those clinical services are delivered at the population level or at the level of families. Chronically ill individuals and their families or other caregivers are particularly likely to benefit from such an emphasis, given the ongoing and often complex therapeutic self-care demands with which they must cope.

In this model, the nurse case manager assesses patient and family strengths and health needs, provides direct care in the form of teaching, delivers a full range of therapeutic nursing interventions, and continually monitors the effectiveness of these interventions. This role includes, but is not limited to, providing a gateway into the health care system, making referrals for health and social services as necessary, and monitoring service utilization for the express purpose of ensuring appropriateness of services. In addition to the direct care, service coordination, individual and family teaching, and advocacy roles described, the full scope of advanced practice nurse case managers should also include prescription of commonly used therapeutic agents, including medications and alternative therapies such as biofeedback, to assist clients with symptom management. Because debilitating symptoms such as pain, nausea, dyspnea, fatigue, anxiety, and depression can interfere with both functional status and quality of life, advanced practice nursing case managers should be prepared to provide a full range of symptom management modalities.

Nurse case managers should provide such care across settings, including clinics, individuals' homes, workplace, hospitals, and subacute care facilities. Again, like their ACNP colleagues, their focus is patient-centered, rather than limited to a particular setting. The work of nurse case managers should include health promotion, primary, secondary, and tertiary illness prevention, service brokering, and education and support of individuals and families within the contexts of their homes and communities. The evolutionary nature of the role lies both in the ability of these individuals to move across settings with patients and in their ability to provide advanced practice nursing services while maximizing system resources on behalf of patients. Thus, the role expansion described here has as its base a population-focused, patient-centered emphasis.

Pharmacologic prescriptive privileges should be extended to advanced practice nurse case managers to cover drugs that are commonly used for *management* of symptoms. Such privileges differ from those of primary or acute care nurse practitioners because they are limited to drugs used for symptom management. We suggest that advanced practice nurses such as nurse case managers can add value to their therapeutic interventions if they are equipped with the capacity to initiate and evaluate the full breadth of these interventions appropriate to their scope of practice. Patients experiencing new comorbidities or whose signs and symptoms indicate serious exacerbations of their primary chronic illnesses should be referred to their primary care provider, much as other advanced practice nurses refer these person when care needs exceed their scopes of practice. The benefits of close monitoring using such strategies include earlier referral, timely responses to exacerbation of illness or symptoms, and effective and efficient use of resources.

Advanced practice nurse case managers might be employed by any community-based health agency, such as home health or outpatient clinics. The role is particularly well suited, however, to vertically integrated systems of care, including, but not limited to, managed care organizations and integrated service delivery networks. The advantage of incorporating advanced practice nurse case managers within these large systems lies in their skill in following clients throughout a system and their patient-centeredness. Increasingly, vertically integrated systems are emphasizing system-wide clinical outcomes, employing nurses with this level of preparation makes it far more likely that such systems will be able to monitor, manage, and enhance systemwide outcomes for chronically ill populations. This is a difficult task at best, within loosely organized community systems composed of numerous autonomous agencies. Advanced practice nurse case managers could work well within such environments, perhaps employed by local health departments or large home health agencies, to advance systemwide goals for clinical outcomes.

In such cases, it would be advantageous for a nurse case manager to facilitate development and implementation of a communitywide coordinating council (Alter & Hage, 1993). Groups such as these would allow for more formal interorganizational cooperation and interdisciplinary care coordination for target populations. For example, community coordinating councils would provide an environment conducive to the development of joint programs for populations with complex needs.

TABLE 13.1 Comparisons Between Acute Care Nurse Practitioners and
Nurse Case Managers

Dimension	Acute Care Nurse Practitioner	Nurse Case Manager
Clinical Focus	• Episodic focus	• Distributive focus
	• Help chronically ill individuals & their families manage an episode of illness; e.g., an exacerbation of a chronic illness or an episode of a new comorbidity.	• Help chronically ill individuals & their families manage health care *over time*, during recovery from acute illness and periods of remission. Emphasis is on health promotion, and primary, secondary, and tertiary prevention related to current and new health problems. Emphasis on managing care within the home and community and partnering with family or other care partners.
Usual Site of Care	• Hospital and transitional sites of care, including subacute care, nursing homes, and client homes during the early recovery period.	• Client homes, clinics, workplaces, and places of worship.
Intervention Strategies	• Diagnosis of common acute exacerbations of chronic illness	• Client and family assessment, including health assessment, and assessment of family health and family dynamics
	• Diagnosis of human responses to acute exacerbation of illness	• Client and family teaching regarding usual health-related self-care and therapeutic self-care
	• Management of acute exacerbation of illness, including prescription of pharmacotherapeutics, patient self-care regimens, and therapeutic self-care education	• Symptom assessment and management, including prescription of pharmacotherapeutics and care regimens

Nurse case managers then, complement the advanced practice nursing services provided by their acute care nurse practitioner colleagues by managing the care of selected target populations over time and across sites of care. Thus, nurse case managers complete the full continuum of care when provided jointly with acute care nurse practitioners. The synergistic linking of both roles advances comprehensive care through systematic extension of advanced practice nursing services across the full spectrum of care environments. Table 13.1 compares the two roles, particularly clinical focus, site of care, and role functions.

Role Complementarity

The interventions used by acute care nurse practitioners and nurse case managers represent a contemporary reformulation of practice to a focus on learning to live with chronic illness to maximize residual health and to ensure that one's life is not defined solely by that illness. This means that *symptom management*, in its fullest sense, rather than symptom monitoring, becomes a major element in care. The World Health Organization definition of health indicates that health is a resource, to be used to make it possible to live life in the ways one prefers. Those with chronic illnesses possess somewhat less of this resource. Thus, if acute care nurse practitioners and nurse case managers function effectively in their complementary roles, residual health can be maintained or enhanced so these individuals and their families can concentrate on the business of living and prevent the development of new health problems. This connotes a focus on health promotion, and primary, secondary, and tertiary illness prevention, including symptom management. If the hallmark of advanced practice nursing is integration of the advances in nursing science into the ongoing work of patient care, it is also evident that nursing science takes on true relevance when applied to the resolution of patient care problems.

Contemporary formulations of advanced practice roles, such as proposed here, are at variance with many interpretations of nursing work. Indeed, the literature regarding the work of nurses, notably some of the nursing administrative literature and a variety of sociological views of nurses' work, use production models of work to explain what nurses actually do and to account for variables that impact patient care delivery (Brannon, 1994). Much of this work analyzes the *structure* of nursing care and examines variables such as those productivity ratios that are based on output rather than outcome models of care (e.g., registered nurse to patient ratios and registered nurse to bed ratios) (Omachonu & Nanda, 1989). Newer practice roles, especially those configured for advanced practice nurses, emphasize the *processes* and *outcomes* of care, as well as the pivotal linkages that provide evidence of the efficacy of nursing intervention for improved clinical outcomes (Lamb, 1995). These conceptualizations of role are based on the notions of Friss (1994), Benner (1994), Tanner and colleagues (1987) in which nursing is described as a practice-based discipline in which elements of theoretical and practice-based knowledge are brought to bear in matters of health and illness and in modification and resolution of patient problems (ANA, 1995; ANA, 1995). Indeed, new administrative paradigms suggest that it is imperative that nursing rethink and reframe not only the work of nursing but also the explanations of nurses' work that they are willing to provide policymakers, purchasers, providers, employers, and consumers.

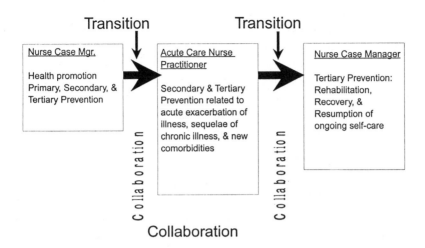

Figure 13.1: Collaborative Relationships Between Acute Care Nurse Practitioners and Nurse Case Managers

Jenkins and Sullivan-Marx (1994) called for establishment of clinical partnerships between primary care nurse practitioners and community-based nurse case managers. This represents the type of partnering and role complementarity that is likely to enhance health system effectiveness. Another logical area for advanced practice nursing role complementarity is between acute care nurse practitioners and nurse case managers. Such complementarity holds special advantages for chronically ill populations, whose members are likely to periodically require acute care services and also require health promotion, and primary, secondary, and tertiary illness prevention. Figure 13.1 depicts a conceptual model of the collaborative relationships described here on behalf of chronically ill populations. Much of the collaboration between nurses in these roles occurs when patients are in transition phases, as nurses consult with one another to help patients and their families manage these transitions. Role collaboration should also be fruitful within particular settings, such as within hospitals or home health agencies. In these cases, acute care nurse practitioners have special knowledge and expertise in the diagnosis and treatment of new comorbidities or development of sequelae of existing chronic illnesses. Nurse case managers, on the other hand, possess special knowledge of these patients and their families because of long-standing relationships with them and know how well they are managing self-care demands and the experience of living with particular symptoms. Furthermore, nurse case managers are experts at managing the health care system to benefit patients within the constraints posed by

financial limitations and reimbursement realities. High levels of clinical benefits may be gained by building structures that articulate the complementarity
between these roles and provide an opportunity to build advanced nursing
practices that are both horizontally and vertically linked, and that provide
chronically ill clients and their families with the experience of seamlessness in
whatever system of care they are participating. Issues of territoriality must be
overcome, however. Also, financial reimbursement structures need to be developed that will reward the boundary-spanning, integrative new roles.

Teaching Role Complementarity

Because acute care nurse practitioners and nurse case managers function in
complementary roles, their educational needs and the strategies to achieve
educational objectives should reflect this complementarity. This means that
both specialties need some common coursework as well as selected coursework
unique to the scope of their practice foci. Both groups aim to help chronically
ill populations achieve the highest level of health possible, targeting Healthy
People 2000 health promotion and illness prevention goals (USDHHS, 1991).

Much of the health promotion and illness prevention efforts of acute care
nurse practitioners emphasize secondary and tertiary prevention, in particular
(although not exclusively). This emphasis suggests that acute care nurse practitioners and nurse case managers need to know how to perform advanced
health assessment of individuals and families, as well as preparation in advanced pharmacology. Both groups should also be prepared to provide nursing
management of symptoms related to chronic illness and to work collaboratively with other health professionals on symptom management problems
(UCSF, 1994). Advanced course work in pharmacology and therapeutics pre-
pares both acute care nurse practitioners and nurse case managers with prescriptive capabilities consistent with the specialty needs of the populations that
they serve. Finally, both groups should be prepared to identify, measure, and
monitor clinical outcomes.

Preparation of ACNPs focuses on high intensity nursing needs of acutely ill
persons, thereby necessitating coursework in pathophysiology and management of acute exacerbations of chronic illnesses. Risk appraisal is a core element
of the ACNP role, consistent with the specialty needs of the chronically ill
patients who characterize high intensity environments. Of particular relevance
is the ability to draw on nursing, as well as the basic and applied sciences, to
think critically, to make inferences, and to translate these into sophisticated
judgments aimed at stabilizing or improving patient health status.

The preparation of nurse case managers involves a unique combination of
clinical and system skills, reflecting their practice emphasis on helping chroni-

cally ill, vulnerable persons meet both clinical and system-related needs. Nurse case managers require preparation in the clinical areas of community and family assessment, care coordination, providing and monitoring therapeutic interventions, and evaluation of outcomes, as well as resource management. The systems emphasis held by nurse case managers is unique with its primary focus on the client and family needs, rather than on staff or organizational needs. Secondary to this client focus, however, is a deep appreciation of the fact that if the context for clinical care disintegrates, then clients lose access to services from at least that particular organization. Thus, nurse case managers hold both a clinical focus on the needs of particular target populations as well as a focus on managing organizational resources (including fiscal, human, and information resources) so that clinical needs are well served over time.

One way to teach role complementarity is to combine nurse case managers and acute care nurse practitioners within those courses that they need in common, thus giving them the opportunity to analyze the ways in which their roles do complement one another and help clients achieve a perception of seamlessness and continuity over time. We propose that the ideal situation is to enroll both groups of students together in selected seminars and to design opportunities for them to work together in clinical practice. These experiences allow them time to critically reflect on how role complementarity works in practice and to develop strategies for maximizing role complementarity.

A collaborative teaching model at the graduate level should include joint seminars in which students actively develop solutions to patient and family problems. The optimal teaching and learning strategy for preparing nurses to fill these roles is one that models complementarity and emphasizes the full scope of services. Such a model will demonstrate how two roles that might initially appear to be competitive are, in fact, complementary and can be actualized through collaborative activity between two categorically different types of advanced nurse providers. Problem-based learning is an ideal teaching strategy for actively engaging students in synthesizing new approaches to patient problems.

An additional strategy for teaching role complementarity is to involve faculty from acute care and community health specialty areas in developing and teaching courses and in student advising. Another strategy for role modeling complementarity and collaboration by faculty is through development of joint faculty practices. Development of viable acute care nurse practitioner and nurse case management collaborative practices provides opportunities for students to participate in joint care planning with faculty, and to jointly develop evaluation strategies for measurement of system-level clinical, organizational, and fiscal outcomes. Such faculty practices also provide a laboratory for engaging students alongside faculty in reimbursement negotiations, thereby further preparing them to assume these evolving roles.

OUTCOMES OF ROLE COMPLEMENTARITY

Symptom management advances are a case in point to illustrate the management of high-intensity patients and the need for ACNPs and NCMs to practice on the edge of innovation. Anticipated outcomes of nurse-based interventions can occur at either or both the client/family or systems levels. In the role reformulations proposed here, it is imperative that acute care nurse practitioners and nurse case managers implement advances in symptom management and that they are prepared to evaluate the effectiveness of these interventions. Advanced practice nurses must engage in data- and evidence-based practice. Advanced practice nurses are held accountable for the direction of change that patient outcomes may take. For example, it is essential that ACNPs and NCMs critically examine what outcomes can be achieved for chronically ill persons in circumstances of deterioration, as well as stabilization and improvement, to improve quality of life, even when cure is not a possible outcome of treatment. ACNPs and NCMs will need to analyze complex data and achieve coordinated services to ensure outcomes.

Client/Family Level

We propose that at the client and family level, there are two types of outcomes: condition-specific and treatment-specific (Fitzpatrick, J., personal communication, June, 1995). Outcomes at the condition-specific level relate to preventing symptom occurrence, reducing or modifying signs and symptoms of illness and disease, and examining the consequences of nursing action under specified conditions and with specified populations who can benefit from treatment generated through delivery of nursing services.

Treatment-specific outcomes at the patient level relate to evaluation of the overall utility of a clinical guideline or practice protocol, for example, or a fine-grained analysis of harms and risks associated with treatment in specified individuals and groups. Both condition and treatment-specific outcomes can be framed from biophysical, behavioral, sociocultural, economic, or spiritual perspectives. Under both sets of outcome conditions (Fields, personal communication, May 1995), the purpose of nurse-based interventions for chronically ill persons or high intensity patients with chronic conditions include a variety of outcomes. Outcomes that result from the synergy created by collaboration between acute care nurse practitioners and nurse case managers are illustrated in Figure 13.2 (Wells, Sebastian, & Walker, 1995).

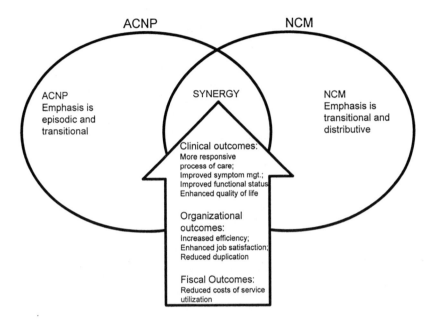

Figure 13.2: Clinical, Organizational, and Fiscal Outcomes of Acute Care Nurse Practitioners and Nurse Case Managers

SOURCE: Modified from Wells, S., Sebastian, J., & Walker, M. K., Issues related to measuring the impact of emerging advanced nursing practice roles. Paper presented to the Tenth Annual Nursing Research Symposium, "Advanced Nursing Practice: Emerging roles and clinical outcomes," University of Chicago Hospitals, Nursing Research, Chicago, Ill., Nov. 17, 1995.

Using population-based surveillance, decision analysis, analysis of patterns of care, and confidence profile methods, the goal is to develop and implement protocols of management that represent treatment-specific outcomes. These protocols of management defy previously determined scopes of provider-specific practices and, ultimately, lead to management of condition-specific interventions. Condition-specific interventions, in turn, set the stage for analysis and feedback in evaluating treatment effectiveness. Finally, outcomes guidelines emerge from these processes, facilitating the clinical benchmarking of best practices and, ultimately, process improvement.

System Level

Incorporation of acute care nurse practitioners and nurse case managers into integrated health care systems has the potential to lead to improved system level outcomes. In one respect, individual and family outcomes are actually system level effects, because of the assumption that chronically ill individuals require services from multiple levels and sources of care (Provan & Milward, 1995). Beyond that, however, vertically integrated systems should enjoy enhanced cost-effectiveness of interventions provided by individual organizational subunits. Greater cost-effectiveness is likely to result from reductions in duplication of efforts and synergy achieved by planning and implementing care across subunits. Furthermore, well-coordinated and individually tailored service packages should result in reduced hospital readmissions, reduction in emergency room use and reduced use of specialty services.

CONCLUSIONS

We conclude that building a model of complementary advanced practice nursing between acute care nurse practitioners and nurse case managers is one potentially effective strategy for managing the long-term care needs of chronically ill individuals and their families. Either informal collaborative relationships between advanced practice nurses in these evolving roles, or formal programs linking both practitioners offer organizational strategies for achieving the benefits of role complementarity. Such a model should be initiated in graduate programs of nursing preparing these practitioners. Components of the model include joint seminars and clinical practice for both groups of students. They also include faculty structures that model the concepts of complementarity and collaboration. The structure we suggest is one in which faculty from traditionally separate clinical areas, such as adult nursing and community health nursing, collaborate on curriculum design, student admissions, course teaching, and program evaluation. Finally, faculty practices in which advanced practice nursing faculty work together in acute care nurse practitioner and nurse case management roles operationalize the concepts of complementarity and collaboration. The benefits to consumers, nurses, and the health care system will accrue from fully functioning and closely integrated emerging and evolving nursing roles. There is much to be gained.

REFERENCES

Aday, L. A. (1993). *At risk in America: The health and health care needs of vulnerable populations in the United States.* San Francisco: Jossey-Bass.

Aday, L. A. (1994). Health status of vulnerable populations. *Annual Review of Public Health, 15,* 487-509.

Agency for Health Care Policy and Research (1995). *Cancer Pain Guidelines.*

Alter, C., & Hage, J. (1993). *Organizations working together.* Newbury Park, CA: Sage.

American Nurses Association. (1994, September). National Nursing Summit: Nurse of the Future. Chicago.

American Nurses Association. (1995a). *A nursing care report card for acute care.* Washington, DC: ANA.

American Nurses Association and American Association of Critical Care Nurses. (1995b). *Standards of clinical practice and scope of practice for the acute care nurse practitioner.* Washington, DC: ANA.

American Nurses Association. (1995c). *Nursing's Social Policy Statement, 1995.* Washington, DC: ANA.

Baker, C., & Stern, P.N. (1993). Finding meaning in chronic illness as the key to self-care. *Canadian Journal of Nursing Research, 25*(2), 23-36.

Benner, P. (1984). *From novice to expert.* Menlo Park, CA: Addison-Wesley.

Bower, K. A. (1992). *Case management by nurses.* Washington, DC: American Nurses Publishing.

Brannon, R. L. (1994). *Intensifying care: The hospital industry, professionalization, and the reorganization of the nursing labor process.* New York: Baywood.

Brooten, D., & Naylor, M. D. (1995). Nurses' effect on changing patient outcomes. *Image: Journal of Nursing Scholarship, 27*(2), 95-99.

Brown, S. A., & Grimes, E. D. (1993). *A meta-analysis of process of care, clinical outcomes, and cost-effectiveness of nurses in primary care roles: Nurse practitioners and certified nurse-midwives.* Washington, DC: American Nurses Publishing.

Clochesy, J. M., Daly, B. J., Idemoto, B. K., Steel, J., & Fitzpatrick, J. J. (1994). Preparing advanced practice nurses for acute care. *American Journal of Critical Care, 3,* 255-259.

Cohen, E. L., & Cesta, T. G. (1993). *Nursing case management: From concept to evaluation.* St. Louis: C.V. Mosby.

Corbin, J. A., & Strauss, A. (1988). *Unending work and care: Managing chronic illness at home.* San Francisco : Jossey Bass.

Department of Health and Human Services, Public Health Service. (1991). *Healthy People 2000: National health promotion and disease prevention objectives.* U.S. Department of Health and Human Services, Public Health service, Pub. No. (PHS) 91-50212, U.S. Government Printing Office, Washington, DC.

Ethridge, P. (1991). A nursing HMO: Carondelet St. Mary's experience. *Nursing Management, 22*(7), 22-27.

Ethridge, P., & Lamb, G. (1989). Professional nursing: Case management improves quality, access, and cost. *Nursing Management, 20*(3), 30-35.

Friss, L. (1994). Nursing studies laid end-to-end form a circle. *Journal of Health Politics, Policy, & Law, 19,* 597-663.

Hall, J. E., & Weaver, B. R. (1977). *Distributive nursing practice: A systems approach to community health.* Philadelphia: J. B. Lippincott.

Jenkins, M. L., & Sullivan-Marx, E. M. (1994). Nurse practitioners and community health nurses: Clinical partnerships and future visions. *Nursing Clinics of North America, 29,* 459-470.

Keane, A., & Richmond, T. (1993). Tertiary nurse practitioners. *Image: Journal of Nursing Scholarship, 25,* 281-284.

Lamb, G. (1995). Case management. In J. Fitzpatrick & J. Stevenson (Eds.), *Annual review of nursing research,* (pp. 117-136). New York: Springer.

Lamb, G. S., & Huggins, D. (1990). The professional nursing network. In G. G. Mayer, M. J. Madden, & E. Lawrenz (Eds.), *Patient care delivery models.* Rockville, MD: Aspen.

Lancaster, J. (1996). The history of community health and community health nursing. In M. Stanhope and J. Lancaster (Eds.), *Community health nursing: Promoting health of aggregates, families, and individuals* (4th ed., pp. 3-20). St. Louis: Mosby-YearBook.

Lancero, A. W., & Gerber, R. M. (1995). Comparing work satisfaction in two case management models. *Nursing Management, 26*(11), 45-48.

Lenz, E., Suppe, F., Gift, A. G., Pugh, L. C., & Milligan, R. A. (1995). Collaborative development of middle-range nursing theories: Toward a theory of unpleasant symptoms. *Advances in Nursing Science, 17*(3), 1-13.

Lumsdon, K. (1994, August 5). Corralling the clinical integration beast. *Hospitals and Health Networks,* 48-49.

Lysaught, J. P. (1970). *An abstract for action.* Report of National Commission for the Study of Nursing and Nursing Education. New York: McGraw-Hill.

National Institute of Nursing Research (1994). Symptom management: Acute pain.

Office of Technology Assessment. (1986). *Nurse practitioners physician assistants and certified nurse midwives: A policy analysis.* Washington, DC.

Omachonu, V. K., & Nanda, R. (1989). Measuring productivity: Outcome vs. output. *Nursing Management, 20*(4), 35-40.

Orem, D. (1985). *Nursing: Concepts of practice.* New York: McGraw-Hill.

Pew Health Professions Commission. (1995). *Critical challenges: Revitalizing the health professions for the twenty-first century.* San Francisco, CA: UCSF Center for the Health Professions.

Provan, K. G., & Milward, H. B. (1991). Institutional-level norms and organizational involvement in a service-implementation network. *Journal of Public Administration Research and Theory, 1,* 391-417.

Provan, K. G., & Milward, H. B. (1995). A preliminary theory of interorganizational network effectiveness: A comparative study of four community mental health systems. *Administrative Science Quarterly, 40,* 1-32.

Safriet, B. J. (1992). Health care dollars and regulatory expense: The role of advanced practice nursing. *Yale Journal of Regulation, 9*(2), 417-487.

Sebastian, J. G. (1994). *Resource, efficiency, and institutional pressures and the structure of cooperative interorganizational relationships in a mental health service delivery network.* Unpublished dissertation: University of Kentucky, Lexington, Ky.

Sebastian, J. G. (1996). Vulnerability and vulnerable populations: An introduction. In M. Stanhope and J. Lancaster (Eds.), *Community health nursing: Promoting health of aggregates, families, and individuals* (4th ed., pp. 623-646). St. Louis: Mosby-YearBook.

Tanner, C., Padrick, K., Westfall, U., Putzier, D. (1987). Diagnostic reasoning strategies of nurses and nursing students. *Nursing Research, 36*(3), 358-363.

The University of California in San Francisco, School of Nursing, Symptom Management Faculty Group. (1994). A model for symptom management. *Image: Journal of Nursing Scholarship, 26,* 272-276.

Van Agthoven, W., & Plomp, H. (1989). The interpretation of self-care: A difference in outlook between clients and home nurses. *Social Science and Medicine, 29,* 245-252.

Walker, M. K. (1995, August 10). Public policy, health care reform, and innovation in nursing practice. American Association of Nurse Anesthetists. 62nd Annual Meeting, Minneapolis, MN.

Wells, S., Sebastian, J., & Walker, M. K. (1995, November 17). *Issues related to measuring the impact of emerging advance nursing practice roles.* Paper presented at the Tenth Annual Nursing Research Symposium, "Advancing nursing practice: Emerging roles and clinical outcomes," University of Chicago Hospitals Nursing Research, Chicago.

Zander, K. (1988). Nursing case management: Strategic management of cost and quality outcomes. *Journal of Nursing Administration, 18*(5), 23-30.

Author Index

Subject index

About the Chairperson/Editor

Diane Gardner Huber, PhD, RN, is an associate professor, College of Nursing, the University of Iowa, where she is one of the core faculty in Nursing Service Administration teaching both graduate and undergraduate students. She specializes in leadership and nursing care management. Dr. Huber also is the Adjunct Director of Nursing at Mercy Hospital, Iowa City, Iowa. This adjunct position is a service-education collaborative position. She is active in a variety of professional nursing organizations, especially the American Organization of Nurse Executives and the American Nurses Association. Dr. Huber has held nursing positions in ambulatory care and acute care. She has been a staff nurse, nurse supervisor, and division director. Her clinical specialty is maternal-child nursing with an emphasis on pediatrics and intensive care nursing. Dr. Huber's research areas are human resources management, nursing administration, and informatics applications, especially a nursing management minimum data set and a management innovations evaluation portfolio, and, second, maternal-child nursing, especially fatigue in postpartum women. Her most recent research projects are related to the development of a management evaluation system, the use of nurse extenders, the development and testing of a nursing management minimum data set, a survey of nursing centers, post-operative vital signs monitoring, and nursing telephone interventions. She has received the American Nurses' Foundation/American Organization of Nurse Executives' Scholar Award (1991), and the 1994 American Organization of Nurse Executives' Research Scholar Award. She has been involved with 15 funded projects, has authored one book, has more than 29 publications, and has done numerous international, national, and local presentations of her work.

209

Sue A. Moorhead, PhD, RN is an assistant professor at the University of Iowa College of Nursing. Dr. Moorhead teaches an overview of nursing courses for beginning nursing students. She also supervises senior students in internship experiences during the final clinical course. In addition, Dr. Moorhead is a Colonel in the U.S. Army Reserve with both active duty and reserve experience. Most recently, she completed assignments as chief nurse in the two U.S. Army reserve hospitals in Iowa. Her research interests focus on the development and implementation of standardized nursing language. She is an investigator on the Nursing Interventions Classification (NIC) team and has developed nursing interventions in the classification. She presently serves as the facilitator for the testing of this classification at Genesis Medical Center in Davenport, Iowa, as part of the current grant. Dr. Moorhead is an investigator on the Nursing Outcomes Classification (NOC) and chairs the group developing outcomes in the psychological and cognitive area. Her current research focuses on mapping nonstandardized nursing data into standardized language using these classifications. She also works with nurses attempting to add standardized languages in both practice and educational settings. This volume is the first to be edited by Dr. Moorhead, who has been a board member for several years.

About the Contributors

Larry Anna Afifi, RNC, PhD, is Nurse Clinician II, Student Health Services, University of Iowa.

Mary Ann Anderson, RN, PhD, is Assistant Professor at the University of Chicago, College of Nursing, Quad Cities Program in Rock Island Illinois.

Constance Burgess, MS, RN, is President of Burgess & Associates in Lakewood, California.

Jeanette Daly, PhD, RN, is Director of Nursing at Greenwood Manor, Iowa City, Iowa.

Boni Johnson, RN, BA, CNA, is Nursing Quality Coordinator at Gundersen Lutheran Medical Center in La Crosse, Wisconsin.

Connie Delaney, PhD, RN is Associate Professor at the College of Nursing, University of Iowa in Iowa City.

Judith Erlen, is associate Professor and Associate Director at the Center for research in Chronic Disorders, University of Pittsburgh School of Nursing.

Ellen Fineout, MS, RN-C, is Advanced Practice Nurse at Strong Memorial Hospital, Rochester, New York.

Denise Fitzgerald, MS, RN-C, is Advanced Practice Nurse at Strong Memorial Hospital, Rochester , New York.

Sally Friend, BSN, MEd, is Nursing Finance and Systems Coordinator at Gundersen Lutheran Medical Center in La Crosse, Wisconsin.

K. Sue Haddock, RN, PhD, is Assistant Professor, College of Nursing, University of South Carolina in Columbia, South Carolina. She is also Nurse Executive, J. F. Byrnes Center for Geriatric Medicine, Education, and Research, South Carolina Department of Mental Health, Columbia, South Carolina.

Rosemary T. Hall, MSN, RN, is Clinical Instructor at the University of Miami School of Nursing in Miami, Florida.

Janet K. Harrison, EdD, RN, is Professor of Nursing at the Hahn School of Nursing, University of San Diego.

Lelia B. Helms, JD, PhD is Professor in the Division of Planning, Policy, and Leadership in the College of Education at the University of Iowa.

Deborah Horst, MS, RN-C, is Advanced Practice Nurse at Strong Memorial Hospital, Rochester, New York.

Dickey Johnson, RN, is Clinical Systems Analyst, Information Services at the Children's Medical Center of Dallas, Texas.

Rita Knight, MS, RN-C, is Advanced Practice Nurse at Strong Memorial Hospital, Rochester, New York.

Joellen Koerner, is Vice President, Patient care at Sioux Valley Hospital in Sioux Falls, South Dakota.

Mary Ellen Kunz, MS, RN-C, is Advanced Practice Nurse at Strong Memorial Hospital, Rochester, New York.

Eileen Lumb, RN, MS, is Advanced Practice Nurse in the Emergency Department at the University of Rochester Medical Center in Rochester, New York.

Julie MacDonald, RN, MS, is Vice President Patient Service at Gundersen Lutheran Medical Center in La Crosse, Wisconsin.

Beth Martin, MS, RN-C, is Advanced Practice Nurse at Strong Memorial Hospital, Rochester, New York.

Peg Mehmert, MSN, RN, is Director, Nursing Practice/Systems Integration, Patient Services Division, Genesis Medical Center, Davenport, Iowa.

Frances Morgan, BSN, RNC, is Clinical manager, Bon Secours Nursing Center, Ellicot City, Maryland.

Lisa Norsen, MS, RN-C, is Clinical Chief, Medical Nursing Practice at Strong Memorial Hospital, Rochester, New York.

Janice Opladen, MS, RN-C, is Advanced Practice Nurse at Strong Memorial Hospital, Rochester, New York.

Richard Redman, PhD, RN, is Associate Professor, Director, Division of Nursing and Health Care Systems Administration Programs, Office of Community partnership, School of Nursing, University of Michigan, Ann Arbor, Michigan.

Ellen Schmidt, MS, RN-C, is Advanced Practice Nurse at Strong Memorial Hospital, Rochester, New York.

Juliann G. Sebastian, PhD, RN, CS, is Associate Professor, Community Health Nursing and Administration Division, Director of Clinical Affairs, University of Kentucky College of Nursing.

Patricia Stahura, MSN, RN, is Director of Nursing, Integrated Health Services at Greenbriar in Miami, Florida.

Ruth M. Tappen, EdD, RN, FAAN, Christine E. Lynn Eminent Scholar, is Professor at Florida Atlantic University College of Nursing in Boca Raton, Florida.

Marian Turkel, MSN, RN, is Assistant Professor at Florida Gulf University in Fort Myers, Florida.

Mary Walker is Professor of Adult Nursing at the University of Kentucky, College of Nursing, Lexington, Kentucky.